# MIGRANT ACADEMICS' NARRATIVES OF PRECARITY AND RESILIENCE IN EUROPE

# Migrant Academics' Narratives of Precarity and Resilience in Europe

*Edited by Olga Burlyuk and Ladan Rahbari*

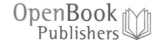

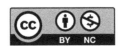 
Digital material and resources associated with this volume are available at https://doi.org/10.11647/OBP.0331#resources.

ISBN Paperback: 978-1-80064-923-1
ISBN Hardback: 978-1-80064-924-8
ISBN Digital (PDF): 978-1-80064-925-5
ISBN Digital ebook (EPUB): 978-1-80064-926-2
ISBN Digital ebook (AZW3): 978-1-80064-927-9
ISBN XML: 978-1-80064-928-6
ISBN HTML: 978-1-80064-929-3
DOI: 10.11647/OBP.0331

Cover image: Filip Kominik, 'Before the Czech' (2017), https://unsplash.com/photos/IHtVbLRjTZU. Cover design: Jeevanjot Kaur Nagpal

# Table of Contents

# Introduction: Narrating Migrant Academics' Precarity and Resilience in Europe

*Ladan Rahbari and Olga Burlyuk*

We started writing this introduction in January 2022, as the world was dealing with ongoing uncertainties caused by the global COVID-19 pandemic. A year before that, in January 2021, we connected with each other in a rather accidental way. We had both published pieces in the *Journal of Narrative Politics*, in which we shared our experiences as migrant academics (Rahbari, 2020; Burlyuk, 2019). It was our shared sense of frustration and the desire to 'tell academic stories'—to tell stories about academics and to tell stories as part of our academic work—that brought us together. Through our conversations, the frustration and a strange sense of familiarity blossomed into something more, and over the course of the following weeks, after we first spoke via email and were restricted by the hurdles of meeting one another under COVID-19 regulations, we met each other online. Our pieces mentioned above on the subject of academic migrants' precarity had by then received a great deal of attention within our academic circles and beyond: not so much academic attention in the form of citations or recognitions, but attention in the form of emotionally inflected emails of support, solidarity, and occasionally of irritation, anger, and curiosity. Through our short autobiographic pieces, we realized we were not only connected to each other but also to a large network of scholars from the 'Global South,' who, in return, shared their stories as migrant academics with us.

 https://doi.org/10.11647/OBP.0331.23

This project was thus built on those narratives and has brought together stories by various migrant academics from the 'Global South' who write about their experiences of precarity and resilience in academia in the 'Global North.' From the 'wandering scholar' (Kim, 2009) and 'stuck and sticky' academics (Tzanakou and Henderson, 2021), academics' mobility has been conceptualized in relation to the internationalization and globalization of the academy and the proliferation of the image of the academic as a neoliberal mobile subject. We have benefited from insightful scholarly works such as Anesa Hosein, Namrata Rao, Chloe Shu-Hua Yeh, and Ian M. Kinchin's edited volume (2018), *Academics' International Teaching Journeys: Personal Narratives of Transitions in Higher Education,* which addresses the personal conflicts and challenges that one encounters through being an international academic. Victoria Reyes's *Academic Outsider: Stories of Exclusion and Hope* shows how academic institutions fail academics from marginalized backgrounds and hence create 'outsiders.' What characterizes this book is our focus on the diasporic precarity of mobile/migrant academics while attempting to extend existing work that has drawn on narratives/autoethnographic approaches to academic migration. Within this foci, we aim to contribute to a growing body of work on critical academic mobilities/migrations.

The narratives in this volume recount different forms and levels of precarity, from hiring practices, sexism, and racism to 'culturally accepted' but problematic divisions of labor in academic spaces. The term 'migrant' has been used throughout this volume to refer to 'South-North' migration (and not 'North-North,' 'North-South,' or 'South-South' migration) unless mentioned otherwise. We do not attempt or intend to define the category of 'South-North migrant,' which represents a vast underlying diversity. Whether it is in the academic formulations of 'Global North/Global South' or in studying the topics of migration and gendered, racial, colored, and other embodied/perceived identities, othering has become part of the process of sense-making. By marking certain bodies as mobile/migrant, the often unnamed and undiscussed immobile subjects are rendered 'normal.' These types of othering in their intersectional forms have been part of (sometimes very well-intentioned) academic inquiries.

We do not believe that a single comprehensive definition of the term 'migrant' is possible at all; instead, we use it broadly in accordance with the self-identification of contributors. In fact, scrutinizing the discursive definition of 'migrant' is one of the objectives of this book. Contributors to the volume have experienced 'migrancy' or 'migranthood' for various reasons and under different circumstances: from political unrest and war, a lack of political freedom, or because they have sought better working and living conditions than the ones in their countries of birth/ stay. Thus, the level of '(in)voluntariness' of the migratory mobility, with all its intricacies, has not impacted the editors' decision to include/ exclude a contribution.

## Precarity and resilience

Academia is not the first area that comes to mind when speaking of precarity. It is often considered a space of knowledge production, status, social prestige, and sometimes—but not always—'progressiveness.' Despite this privileged access to status, academics are not immune to precarity, as systematic powerlessness is distributed along all social strata, including the academic context (Zheng 2018). Precarity has been presented as a state of being for many and a condition of our times— where we are experiencing the weakening of welfare states, the growth of neoliberal social order and economies, climate change, and the recent pandemic-induced state of precarity.

The academy's current state is precarious for many reasons, including job insecurity, scarcity of positions, insular community, unpaid work, unhealthy working conditions, the inadequacy of commitment to anti-discrimination, and lack of academic freedom (Urbanaviciute et al., 2021; Ahmed, 2004; Beban and Trueman, 2018; Bosanquet, Mantai, and Fredericks, 2020; Roth and Vatansever, 2020) within a neoliberal context that promotes self-care instead of solidarity, individualizes responsibility, masks inequalities, and pathologizes radical thinking about change (Rahbari, 2021; Barclay, 2021). In addition, Eurocentrism in academia leads to the (re)reproduction of inequalities in the formulation and dissemination of knowledge (Rahbari, 2015). This makes academic conditions particularly precarious for migrant academics (Sang and Calvard, 2019), especially for those with ambiguous (legal) status, as the loss of previously built social networks and various forms of discrimination and disadvantage impact their lives as *academics* and as *migrants*.

Coupled with the rampant neoliberal and competition-based work culture in academic spheres in the 'Global North,' inequality materializes in diverse forms in academia. Discrimination based on gender, race, ability, and age—among other factors—has been shown to affect everyday life, the physical and mental health of academics, and 'survival' within an academic system that is often characterized by individualism and hierarchical relations (Bhopal, 2018; Vatansever, 2020; Wekker, 2016; Ryan-Flood and Gill, 2009). Academia inherits the flaws of the larger social system in which it is embedded. As Cecilia Ridgeway (2014) puts it, the Western labor market is only 'ostensibly meritocratic.' The narratives in this volume expose the intersectional effects of the discrimination mentioned above on the everyday lives, career paths, mental health, and life course trajectories of migrant academics.

Precarity has already been used to analyze how the current state of affairs in the academy contributes to systematic discrimination and molds academic careers into tools of alienation (Zheng, 2018; Adsit et al., 2015) and to answer the question of whether precarity can serve as a critical concept for challenging social exclusions or forming new political collectivities (Zembylas, 2019). We draw on how (feminist) scholarship has taken up precarity as a concept to illustrate different forms of structurally induced and individually perpetuated and suffered powerlessness (Flores Garrido, 2020; Zembylas, 2019; Shildrick, 2019). We extend this structural and lived experience of powerlessness to the realm of academia by centering on autoethnographic and autobiographic insights, and thereby also proliferating accounts of precarity, creating more dialogue around it. In this collection, we illustrate that precarity is not a set of fixed conditions but a complex and multidimensional state that is context-dependent, relational, relative, material, and embodied.

Resilience refers to strategies of endurance that people adopt to facilitate their day-to-day living but which do not really change the circumstances which make their lives difficult (MacLeavy, Fannin, and Larner, 2021). It can be related to how individuals and societies adapt to externally imposed change. Some argue that, even if we cannot change the world, we can survive better by knowing how to adapt (Joseph, 2013). Resilience is a currently debated concept, especially because it has expanded to include neoliberal subjectivities through its use within discourses of self-help and self-improvement (Cretney, 2014). Neoliberalism is understood here as a rationality of government performed through regimes of subjectification that extend the logic of the market—and, specifically, the principles of competition and inequality—to all spheres of human activity (Mavelli, 2019). In this view, resilience becomes a normative concept, an ideal type of human agency fit for the neoliberal logic (Chandler, 2016). However, there is a post-neoliberal discourse on resilience as well, which opens up the possibility for resilience to be conceptualized in a way where individuals are not mere targets of top-down or bottom-up frameworks of government, but contextually empowered selves in a constant process of learning (Mavelli, 2019). In the latter view that we adopt, resilience may have the potential to enable survival and help subjects to learn and prepare for uncertainties and challenges in the future.

Resilience is, however, not experienced in the same way by all people, because our individual vulnerabilities constitute our 'un-freedoms' or the restrictions—material or ideological—that prevent us from adapting to change (Chandler, 2016). Not everyone is afforded the same level of resilience, and scholarly literature has already revealed the gendered and racial nature of resilience (Jakubowicz et al., 2017; Smyth and Sweetman, 2015). Adapting to change, resisting structural challenges, and preparing for future uncertainties is difficult in the presence of inequality, precarity and the shortage or lack of support systems. Different narratives of this book highlight exactly this: that the capacity to become resilient is not distributed equally.

## Why narratives?

We have heard too many times from our students that much of the current teaching and literature on migration takes away the 'humanity' of the subjects, sometimes by overtheorizing and other times through what has come to be accepted as 'conventional' academic writing, which turns migrants into aliens—otherized and unimaginable entities. Narratives occupy a small part of teaching and research into migration and are more often represented in press and journalistic pieces. Autoethnographic and autobiographic work that has been published on migration, otherness, and academia (notably, Shahram Khosravi's *The Illegal Traveller*; Yassir Morsi's *Radical Skin, Moderate Masks*; Paul Carter's *Translations, an Autoethnography*; Ellis Hurd's *The Reflexivity of Pain and Privilege*; Nicola Mai's *Mobile Interventions*; Daniel Nettle's *Hanging on to the Edges*) is rare. It is unconventional to use narratives for academic data gathering and analysis, and the 'objectivity' and academic viability of these sources is questioned. Even when diversity, intersectionality, and decolonization are seemingly promoted, and alterity is celebrated, as José Esteban Muñoz argued, non-conventional critical work is not validated in all the aspects of the institutional matrix of the academy (Muñoz, 1996b). In fact, the first proposal for this volume was rejected by an academic publisher partly on the grounds that it was not 'academic' enough. Social scientists working with narratives would relate to our experience of being made to defend storytelling as a method of scientific inquiry.

Nonetheless, biographical methods are useful for challenging (at times tacit) assumptions of research on migration (Erel, 2007). The use of narratives and storytelling is a valuable educational resource in teaching settings, as it encourages critical thinking by facilitating students' knowledge of migration (Svendsen et al., 2021). Critical storytelling is crucial to the study of migration, as it contributes to an anti-racist pedagogy in which the otherized speak for themselves (Aveling, 2001). Like critical theories, critical storytelling does not hide behind a pretense of moral and political neutrality (Barone, 1992). This volume has been co-created precisely to tell political stories on migration; similar to Erwin (2021), our stories aim to complicate, disrupt, and make a mess out of discriminatory hegemonic narratives of migration. We refuse to keep implicit the roles and imagery ascribed to migrant academics from the 'Global South' in the 'Global North' academy.

The chapters of this book are born out of migrant academics' interactions and from our conviction that stories connect readers to each other in intimate and relatable ways. We have, therefore, taken up a methodological focus on narratives and autoethnographic accounts of migration. We aimed for this volume to normalize the 'unconventionality' of storytelling in academic publishing. We do not attempt to represent all accounts of precarity or to make claims about *how* autoethnographic and autobiographic methods should be used in academic writing.

Chapters of this book bring elements of creative and experimental writing and narrative-based approaches into the academic sphere. By prioritizing accessibility and relatability, we have decided not to centralize the 'literary value' of the narratives and avoid overly formal language. Both editors have had many conversations with students and colleagues about the problem of accessibility of academic texts. We are well aware that this is a topic that divides academics. Many scholars whose work has been globally read and widely appreciated employ academic language that is not necessarily accessible to the non-expert public. We do not intend to problematize the more conventional modes of academic writing, as others have skillfully done before us (PARISS Collective, 2020), yet we too see space and opportunity in exploring creative, innovative, experimental, aesthetic writing as a way to rethink international social sciences and expand our readership. This is why various contributions in this book are written in different and creative narrative, prose, or poetry formats rather than adhering to conventional academic style and jargon. We hope that this makes the volume readable and accessible to a broader audience than usual (i.e., not just academics and policymakers).

Besides the structural, material, and cultural inequalities and different levels of intersectional powerlessness, individually perceived, embodied, felt, and lived experiences are full of insights into context-specific precarity. Intersectionality is useful in understanding the effects of structural and systematic social conditions on individual lives (Crenshaw, 2017), but even for those people who are located at the same crossroads and experiencing the weight of similar axes of social difference, the experiences of precarity and power will not be the same. While we acknowledge the structural nature of inequalities in cultural, social, and material forms, we believe that individual narratives that connect the elements of history, context, and life stories have the potential to give us an in-depth understanding of precarity and resilience. We are, therefore, in agreement with scholars who have argued that getting a sense of precarity requires 'the art of noticing,' driven by curiosity and based on one's commitment to observation, fieldwork, and slowing down (Tsing, 2015). We also agree that using embodied experiences of power as the basis of knowledge requires writing that is 'animated by the everyday' (Ahmed, 2016). And so, in this book, we step away from conventional academic writing and adopt autobiographic and autoethnographic narratives as a core method of scholarly analysis and reasoning.

## Decolonization and the 'South-North' binary

The narratives in this book will, without a doubt, be perceived by some as provocative and radical. Decolonization cannot occur without hurting feelings, and it cannot be whitewashed. We aim to decolonize the discourses around academic mobility in this book by highlighting the experiences of precarity, resilience, and care in the academic margins. The chapters do not use the term 'decolonization' in the same way (or at all) nor do they refer to it as a singular way of thinking and working within the academy. Decolonization has been used in different chapters to refer to different aspects of the ongoing debates and efforts. As Mamdani (2016) discusses, decolonization has different aspects: the political aspect entails the independence of colonized societies from external domination and broader transformations of institutions, especially those critical to the reproduction of racial and ethnic subjectivities legally enforced under colonialism; the economic aspect consists of local ownership over local resources and the transformation of internal and external institutions that sustain unequal colonial-type economic relations; and the epistemological aspect takes issue with categorizations that are made, unmade, and remade, and thereby apprehend the world. Decolonization involves delinking from the coloniality of power: the reconstruction and the restitution of silenced histories, repressed subjectivities, subalternized knowledges, and languages (Mignolo, 2007). As Gurminder Bhambra (2014) has argued, the colonial matrix of power in the form of two rhetorics of modernity and coloniality has to be central to any discussion of contemporary global inequalities and the historical basis of their emergence.

There has been a critique of the tokenistic usage of the term and its overly ambitious nature when referring to the institutional response to advancing Indigenous achievement in the academy (Cote-Meek and Moeke-Pickering, 2020). Decolonization is sometimes used as a metaphor and superficially adopted into social sciences to reconcile settler guilt and complicity (Tuck and Yang, 2012). Inspired by Davies et al. (2003), our claim of decolonization of migrant academic narratives is based on our contributors reclaiming the discourse on mobility, migration, and precarity, as well as their narratives questioning the predominant neocolonial, gendered, and racial paradigms. This book is a space for the voices of (diasporic) scholars who mainly come from formally or informally colonized contexts from the 'Global South.' They come from 'the asshole of the world,' as Larissa Pelúcio (2014) provocatively calls it; they then moved to the head (the brain), where powerful academic institutions are located, in the 'Global North.' This metaphor illustrates geopolitics that transform certain people into suppliers of data and experiences and others into experts and exporters of theories to be applied and reaffirmed (Pereira, 2019; Connell, 2020). The narratives of this book subvert this logic by placing the experiences and theories in one place: the 'asshole.'

By exploring migration narratives, we would like to showcase the multifacetedness and diversity of migrant experiences. The narratives complicate the assumption that mobility is a privileged state by using migrant academics' experiences of hybrid identity, embodied differences, and marginalization. Even from the start, mobility is not a privilege for the people in the 'Global South,' refugees, displaced people, and (self-)exiled academics. Mobility can cause the loss of different forms of capital, deprive individuals of their care networks, burden them with emotional challenges and loneliness, and expose them to discrimination and othering (Rahbari, 2018; Djundeva and Ellwardt, 2020). While not defining migration in a singular way, the chapters of this book explore the effects of migranthood and mobility, and reflect on the questions of 'voluntary' and 'involuntary' mobility from the 'Global South' to the 'Global North' within the academic context. The complexity of the narratives helps us realize an important objective in the study of migration: the bridging of the dichotomous divide between the study of 'voluntary' and 'forced' migration (de Haas, 2021). They reflect on how we understand 'migrant' subjects and 'migrancy' as a state of being, not only by showing various forms of precarity but also by reflecting on the diversity of ways mobility is practiced and experienced, as well as the mobile subjects' resilience, agency, resistance in implicit or explicit forms, and/or activism.

We have so far continuously used quotation marks to refer to the categories of 'Global South' and 'Global North.' Before dropping the quotation marks, we would like to clarify that, like other scholars (e.g., Andrea Wolvers, 2015; Laura Trajber Waisbich et al., 2021), we find these terms at times useful and, at other times, inadequate and misleading. Choosing terminologies that mark vast geographical locations with different histories is not easy. None of the existing binary formulations—such as center/periphery, West/Orient, rich/poor, and developed/underdeveloped—do justice to the present diversities on each side precisely because of binarization. There are multiple problems with using these concepts, including the connotations of terms used, the inherent binarism in the formulation, and the artificial grouping of multiple and different countries under one category. We decided to leave the terminology choices to the contributors, who have chosen different terminologies to refer to global and international hierarchies in the academy and the world's economic and political order. This decision was based on the diversity of disciplinary backgrounds of the contributors and their consequent preferences for terminologies referring to global geopolitical inequalities.

We, the editors, decided to choose the terms Global South and Global North for ourselves. This is not a perfect choice, but these terms have at least been accepted as non-static concepts with geopolitical shifts, not only concerning the meaning of the terms but also with regard to which countries are considered to be part of the Global South and which the Global North (Wolvers, 2015). South-North migration is defined broadly, not as a strict dichotomy, but as a set of specific cultural, political, or social geographies analytically used to distinguish between forms of migration that entail moving between countries that occupy similar positions in the world's historically created politico-economic hierarchy. This includes movements from countries worldwide (from European peripheries and semi-peripheries) to Western Europe. We aim to address the struggles of these academics who, because of the supposed added prestige of their academic 'upgrade' by moving to the Global North and their relative mobility, may be perceived as more 'privileged' when compared to their fellow academics in the Global South, but always occupy an 'in between' space when it comes to predominantly white academic spaces in the Global North. The volume's contributors problematize the assumptions of 'upward' mobility that rely on the colonial history of knowledge production that imagines the Global North as the core where 'better,' if not 'true,' knowledge is produced (Akena, 2012) and migrant academics are seen as labor migrants of corporate universities.

Yet, while we hope to have attempted to *do* decolonization, we cannot claim to *be* completely decolonized, as we believe that decolonization must be seen as a perpetual project. Besides this, many of us—editors and authors—are currently located in institutions in the Global North, and (either now or throughout our lives) have benefited from the politics of our locations (Rich, 1984) and the consequences of settler colonialism. Some of us are closely connected to geographies of power, wealth, and authority, while others remain deprived of access to powerful affiliations, locations, and institutions.

## Ethical considerations

Without any claims of comprehensive coverage or proportional representation of either the Global South or the Global North, it is worth emphasizing that the pool of lived experiences that the authors' narratives tap into and draw from is diverse. This book does not specifically aim to contribute to debates about diversity in the academy or the lack thereof, but it strives to be a diverse space. The volume's contributors represent different geographies and academic spaces, both in terms of their respective 'birth' or 'stay' countries and in terms of the countries/academic institutions in the Global North that have employed them during part of (or throughout) their academic careers. Both of the editors of this volume are migrant academics too (from Iran and Ukraine) and have our own personal experiences with the subject of precarity in academia. We find it ironic that, on the one hand, the promotion of 'diversity' and hiring of people like 'us' is adopted by universities, assuming that previously excluded groups desire to be a part of mainstream institutions and that everyone will benefit from this inclusion (de Oliveira Andreotti et al., 2015), but on the other hand, when those same people raise problems of racism, sexism, ableism, and structural discrimination at the university, their voices are ignored, if not suppressed. This book is thus a collection of those outcries. And it has been our editorial decision to include a higher number of shorter narratives rather than a smaller number of longer ones, in order to amplify more voices within this volume.

We have aimed to be diverse in contributors' voices in terms of academic disciplines, academic rankings, and countries/regions academics use to tell their 'origin' stories. To accomplish this, we solicited contributions from scholars representing a wide range of disciplines in social sciences and humanities. Likewise, 'seniority' and academic credentials have not been a criterion for contribution. Our contributors occupy different positions in their respective institutions, ranging from early and nearly finished doctoral candidates to early and mid-career academics. The narratives of this book go further by showing how the normalization of hierarchies in academic institutions can fuel, if not directly cause, discrimination and abuse. They address already known forms of precarity based on race, gender, age, ability, religion, nationality, and other intersectional experiences that do not neatly fit within the already known and more extensively researched identification categories.

We are well aware that while diversity is needed to provide opportunities for racialized and minorized students and academics, without structural change, diversity will not go a long way (Arshad et al., 2021). The precarity that the contributors to this book speak of will not change due to their contributions, and their migrancy and embodied differences will remain pathologized. But with the interdisciplinarity and the diversity of themes centered around this precarity, we hope that the volume will also appeal to those housekeeping and maintaining the Master's House (Lorde, 2003), such as diversity officers, managers, and other key decision-makers in the university who can create change on the structural level.

As we and our contributors constructed or recounted our narratives, many ethical dimensions arose, including anonymity, positionality, and reflections on the limitations of 'precarity' as one framework to capture all the diversities, dimensions, and levels of precariousness. With our contributors, we did our utmost best to protect the identities of others who may be implicated in personal accounts without taking away from the authenticity of the narratives. We have adhered to the principles of decolonial feminist scholarship, which advocate for the indigenization of spaces and approaches to scholarship that naturalize and normalize indigenous perspectives and worldviews within the academy (Tuhiwai Smith, 2012) although it is not always easy to step out and away from internalized colonial frameworks of knowledge.

Additionally, from the start of this project, we firmly believed that it was essential that this book be published open access. While open-access publishing democratizes access to content, academic readers will know the appeal of publishing with 'prestigious' academic publishing companies. Academic 'prestige' is closely tied to an institution's symbolic and cultural capital, which in turn often results from economic and political capital. However, some of the publishing practices of these same powerful institutions have led to the perpetuation of unequal access to books and other academic content. We question various structures of power and discrimination in contemporary academia in this book, including the commercial institution of academic publishing as its integral element. Moreover, perhaps the most obvious, immediate, and urgent readership of this book—migrant academics across the globe and across disciplines—is precisely the demographic that often finds itself in precarious situations (including financially) and, therefore, might not be able to afford to buy the book should it be sold commercially. This, in turn, would greatly undermine the spirit of collectivity and solidarity in which this book has been written—and which it aims to strengthen and promote.

## The composition of this book

This book is a carefully curated collection of narrative essays divided into six sections, each consisting of different chapters. The narrative chapters/sections are complemented by this introduction and a final reflection chapter. The distribution of narratives is based on some of the central themes the chapters cover, but there is certainly a level of arbitrariness in this distribution: each of the narratives could be situated rightfully within two or more sections. Therefore, we encourage readers to consider our categorization as a merely descriptive and subjective practice, which they should go beyond.

In the first section of the volume, '(non)belonging,' Vera Axyonova, Sanam Roohi, and Mihnea Tănăsescu reflect on different ways they (do not) belong in the European academy. In Chapter 1, Vera Axyonova regards academic precarity as non-belonging and delves into personalized multidimensional non-belonging experiences. Reviewing her journey from her home country, Kazakhstan, to German academia, Vera raises issues of othering and foreignness, asymmetric power relations, and illusory diversity in Global North universities. Sanam Roohi writes about her experience as a first-generation university graduate from a minority background in India in Chapter 2. Sanam reflects upon her academic trajectory in Amsterdam and in German academia. The chapter contemplates the post-colonial predicament of non-belonging and the embodied negotiations she continues to make as a temporary job-holder and a part of the growing international academic precariat. In Chapter 3, Mihnea Tănăsescu explores how migrant academics are trained to think of their place within the profession and society writ large. The chapter proposes that, despite the academy's proclaimed pledge to diversity and interdisciplinarity, allegiance to one origin and one disciplinary model is routinely requested, performed, and internalized. Consequently, in finding one's own way, one must pass through a continuous process of unlearning.

In the second section, '(in)visible inclusions and exclusions,' Norah Kiereri, Martina Vitáčková, Dragana Stojmenovska, and an anonymous contributor engage with the ways in which borderings and modes of inclusion and exclusion in the academy are rendered (in)visible, and how invisible precarity is ignored and stigmatized. In Chapter 4, Norah Kiereri reflects on the (in)visibility of death in a European city during the COVID-19 pandemic. She recounts her own experience of the painful death of a loved one while working in Europe and the somewhat perplexing reactions (or lack thereof) from her institution and colleagues in the academy. Martina Vitáčková compares the imaginary wall of ice in the Game of Thrones (TV series) to the Iron Curtain still dividing Europe in Chapter 5. She argues that it is close to impossible to penetrate this wall, and even once one is in, one is still considered a wildling. Martina traces this dynamic within academia. Dragana Stojmenovska's narrative in Chapter 6 revolves around how academics are expected to be mobile, yet this mobility is expected differently from academics, depending on their academic and social backgrounds. The chapter is about the day Dragana stopped being an immigrant and not the day she stopped being mobile. Dragana discusses how one is in need of 'permission' even to define oneself, let alone to engage with the country one lives in critically. In Chapter 7, the anonymous author gives their perspective on the challenges of navigating Western academia as an immigrant while having mental health condition(s), all the while being subjected to the rather unforgiving culture of continuous assessment in the new workplace and bearing the extra burden posed by mental illness.

In the following section, 'borders, mobility, and academic 'nomadism,' Maryna Shevtsova, Vjosa Musliu, and Tara Asgarilaleh address the consequences, rewards, and challenges of being mobile academics. Maryna Shevtsova explores a hybrid identity of an early-career female researcher in Western academia dealing with internationalization in Chapter 8. Questioning how one's gender, ethnicity, sexuality, and institutional affiliation intersect, this chapter reflects on how identities are constructed and maintained and how uneven distribution of opportunity structures for mobility among geopolitical spaces and social groups impacts one's self-identity and life chances. Vjosa Musliu shows in Chapter 9 how a lack of hospitality is normalized in the visa application procedures of Western European countries. Vjosa shows the impossibility of British hospitality in its visa procedures for nationals of the Global South. Walking the reader through a personal Kafkaesque visa procedure, Vjosa reveals how British hospitality is regulated by governmentality and surveillance. Tara Asgarilaleh's narrative in Chapter 10 addresses the position of a 'migrant academic' who has to deal with visa applications, a sort of bureaucratic madness that affects the most precarious passports. Tara's chapter unravels the precarity inherent in certain passports and how these passports impact mobile academics despite the invisibility of their precariousness.

The next section of the volume, 'the complexities of privilege and precarity,' engages with the complexity of academic experiences at the intersection of multiple categories of difference through chapters by Apostolos Andrikopoulos, Karolina Kluczewska, Bojan Savić, and Alexander Strelkov. In Chapter 11, Apostolos Andrikopoulos's narrative explores his understanding of race throughout his life; and his racialization as 'white' after moving to the Netherlands as an academic. He asks how appropriate it is to apply the category of 'white' to migrant scholars whose pathway to academia started where whiteness had a different meaning or was less significant as a marker of privilege. Karolina Kluczewska's narrative in Chapter 12 revolves around her experience of joining Tajik academia, referring to the issues of mistrust, mutual favors, and the culture of mediocrity. Karolina discusses how, as she was confronted with new academic conventions and practices, Tajik academia made her question her own positionality in the academy of the Global North. Bojan Savić's narrative in Chapter 13 explores the normalization of his own vulnerability and immigrant otherness through a subjectivity of hope and aspiration. In particular, he embeds the problematization of and ability to cope with precarity in discourses of aspirational temporality and de-territorialized hope for happiness. In Chapter 14, Alexander Strelkov turns to metaphysical explanations to explain why his academic career is so insecure and challenging. The author indulges in an intimate conversation with Saint Precario to reflect upon his own professional and personal Odyssey.

The following three contributions are part of the section 'gendered precarity and sexualization.' In this section, Aslı Vatansever, Emanuela Mangiarotti, and Olga Burlyuk reflect on different aspects of gendered precarity. Aslı Vatansever reflects on gender inequality, hierarchy, and foreignness as an exiled female researcher in European academia in Chapter 15. Given her own conflicting feelings and actions during and after a sexual assault in an academic context, the author confronts the predicaments of resistance and the discrepancies between the theory and practice of feminist solidarity. Emanuela Mangiarotti's narrative in Chapter 16 centers on how the effort to re-integrate into academia in Italy has been chiefly defined by her identity as a homecoming Italian female researcher and how moving 'back' has made her radically aware of the way gender marks endemic precarity within Italian academia. In Chapter 17, Olga Burlyuk walks down memory lane and recollects her professional interactions at the intersection of gender and ethnicity, spanning fifteen years, offering an elaborate sketch of everyday sexism and gendered racism in academia.

In the final section, 'embodied differences and (non)whiteness,' Lydia Namatende-Sakwa, Atamhi Cawayu, Sama Khosravi Ooryad, and Ladan Rahbari reflect on what it means to navigate the European academy while embodying (visible) differences. In Chapter 18, Lydia Namatende-Sakwa recounts her encounters with racism, interweaved with feelings of guilt for leaving her family, and paints a picture of precariousness informed by identity markers of race, sex, and class. In Chapter 19, Atamhi Cawayu illustrates his experiences as a researcher of color in Belgium committed to anti-racism in majority-white academic spaces. The chapter reflects on the challenges of BIPOC academics to shift the academy towards an anti-racist space. Sama Khosravi Ooryad recounts some exclusionary moments and her positionality in the academy as a 'strategic outsider' in Chapter 20. Sama shares examples from her time as a GEMMA student in the Netherlands to illustrate how and why she perceives a need to be alert to exclusions and be critical of toxicities encountered within and beyond Western academia. Ladan Rahbari's narrative in Chapter 21 reflects on academics' performative work and microaggressions in conference rooms and other spaces, and the stark differences between those performances and what happens in more private spaces.

The final essay in the volume is one that reflects on and makes sense of the complexity of the narratives within this volume. In this chapter, Umut Erel discusses the value of collecting and validating stories and how narratives make valuable interventions by challenging exclusions and hierarchies in European academia. She also shares experiences of encounters with gendered and racialized discourses in the academy and how she has been inspired by what she calls 'the killjoy work' of scholars such as Sara Ahmed in making visible and challenging the existing power relations.

## Final words

As you embark on this reading journey, keep in mind that writing the narratives of this book has been a difficult, emotionally taxing, and demanding practice for some of us and exhilarating, empowering, and healing for others. To paraphrase Sara Ahmed (2016), the academy is something we, migrant academics, work *on* as well as *at*. We thank all the contributors for doing the intellectual, emotional, and political work of sharing their narratives in this volume. The act of documenting critical autoethnography and autobiography from the margins is, in itself, precarious work. At the same time, writing about one's precarity is also an exercise in—and a manifestation of—resilience. One of the contributors to this volume wrote their narrative literally overnight. Another one wrote theirs during sick leave taken to preempt burnout.

This book was conceived and actualized in a world saturated with uncertainties and anxieties, including those caused by the COVID-19 global pandemic. As we worked on this collection, Russia launched a full-out war on Ukraine, and the 'Woman, Life, Freedom' uprising arose in Iran, the editors' respective countries. Just like the lives of the contributors to this collection, ours remain entangled with those of people and lands in the Global South. Some of us live with feelings of uprootedness, otherization, longing, and hope, and occupy in-between spaces in the Global North academy as we deal with anxieties of mobility and belonging. Some authors we invited to contribute to the book, all of whom were migrant academics, had to withdraw their contributions precisely because of their already existing precarity or new challenges they faced due to the pandemic or other social, economic, or political realities. Others kindly declined the invitation to contribute, confessing that writing a truthful autobiographical account would require more openness and publicity than they were ready to offer.

The fact that many of those voices are missing in this book is a reminder that precarity has always been and will continue to be a part of academic work, including this book, and that the decolonization achieved by this collective work is a fraction of a step towards the greater challenge of decolonizing migrant academics' narratives. We hope that the narratives of this book will shed some light on the intersectional lived experiences of migrant academics and their genealogy, and perhaps inspire some to find ways to resist the structural and cultural forces perpetuating them.

# Works cited

Janelle Adsit, Sue Doe, Marisa Allison, Paula Maggio and Maria Maisto, 'Affective activism: Answering institutional productions of precarity in the corporate university,' *Feminist Formations* 27/3 (2015): 21–48. https://doi.org/10.1353/ff.2016.0008

Sara Ahmed, 'Declarations of whiteness: The non-performativity of anti-racism,' *Borderlands* 3/2 (2004): 1–54.

Sara Ahmed, *Living a Feminist Life* (Duke University Press, 2016). https://doi.org/10.1215/9780822373377

Francis Adyanga Akena, 'Critical analysis of the production of Western knowledge and its implications for Indigenous knowledge and decolonization', *Journal of Black Studies* 43/6 (2012): 599–619. https://doi.org/10.1177/0021934712440448

Muminah Arshad, Rachel Dada and Cathy Elliott et al., 'Diversity or decolonization? Searching for the tools to dismantle the 'master's house', *London Review of Education* 19/1 (2021): 1–18. https://doi.org/10.14324/LRE.19.1.19

Nado Aveling, "Where do you come from?': Critical storytelling as a teaching strategy within the context of teacher education', *Discourse: Studies in the Cultural Politics of Education* 22/1 (2001): 35–48. https://doi.org/10.1080/01596300120039740

Katie Barclay, *Academic Emotions: Feeling the Institution* (Cambridge University Press, 2021). https://doi.org/10.1017/9781108990707

Thomas E. Barone, 'Beyond theory and method: A case of critical storytelling', *Theory into Practice* 31/2 (1992): 142–146.

Alice Beban and Nicolette Trueman, 'Student workers: The unequal load of paid and unpaid work in the neoliberal university', *New Zealand Sociology* 33/2 (2018): 99–131.

Gurminder K. Bhambra, 'Postcolonial and decolonial dialogues', *Postcolonial Studies* 17/2 (2014): 115–121. https://doi.org/10.1080/13688790.2014.966414

Kalwant Bhopal, *White Privilege: The Myth of a Post-Racial Society* (Policy Press, 2018). https://doi.org/10.2307/j.ctt22h6r81

Agnes Bosanquet, Lilia Mantai, and Vanessa Fredericks, 'Deferred time in the neoliberal university: Experiences of doctoral candidates and early career academics', *Teaching in Higher Education* 25/6 (2020): 736–749. https://doi.org/10.1080/13562517.2020.1759528

Olga Burlyuk, 'Fending off a triple inferiority complex in academia: An autoethnography', *Journal of Narrative Politics* 6/1 (2019): 28–50.

Paul Carter, *Translations, an Autoethnography: Migration, Colonial Australia and the Creative Encounter* (Manchester University Press, 2021).

David Chandler, 'Debating neoliberalism: The exhaustion of the liberal problematic' in David Chandler and Julian Reid, *The Neoliberal Subject: Resilience, Adaptation and Vulnerability* (Rowman & Littlefield Publishers, 2016): 9–16.

Raewyn Connell, *Southern Theory: The Global Dynamics of Knowledge in Social Science* (Routledge, 2020). https://doi.org/10.4324/9781003117346

Sheila Cote-Meek and Taima Moeke-Pickering, *Decolonizing and Indigenizing Education in Canada* (Canadian Scholars' Press, 2020).

Kimberlé W. Crenshaw, *On Intersectionality: Essential Writings* (The New Press, 2017).

Raven Cretney, 'Resilience for whom? Emerging critical geographies of socio-ecological resilience', *Geography Compass* 8/9 (2014): 627–640. https://doi.org/10.1111/gec3.12154

Hein de Haas, 'A theory of migration: The aspirations-capabilities framework', *Comparative Migration Studies* 9/1 (2021): 8. https://doi.org/10.1186/s40878-020-00210-4

Vanessa de Oliveira Andreotti, Sharon Stein, Cash Ahenakew, and Dallas Hunt, 'Mapping interpretations of decolonization in the context of higher education', *Decolonization: Indigeneity, Education & Society* 4/1 (2015): 21–40.

Maja Djundeva and Lea Ellwardt, 'Social support networks and loneliness of Polish migrants in the Netherlands', *Journal of Ethnic and Migration Studies* 46/7 (2020): 1281–1300. https://doi.org/10.1080/1369183X.2019.1597691

Umut Erel, 'Constructing meaningful lives: Biographical methods in research on migrant women', *Sociological Research Online* 12/4 (2007): 35–48. https://doi.org/10.5153/sro.1573

Kira Erwin, 'Storytelling as a political act: Towards a politics of complexity and counter-hegemonic narratives', *Critical African Studies* 13/3 (2021): 237–252. https://doi.org/10.1080/21681392.2020.1850304

Natalia Flores Garrido, 'Precarity from a feminist perspective: A note on three elements for the political struggle', *Review of Radical Political Economics* 52/3 (2020): 582–590. https://doi.org/10.1177/0486613420906930

Anesa Hosein, Namrata Rao, Chloe Shu-Hua Yeh, Ian M. Kinchin (eds), *Academics' International Teaching Journeys: Personal Narratives of Transitions in Higher Education* (Bloomsbury, 2018). https://doi.org/10.5040/9781474289801

Ellis Hurd, *The Reflexivity of Pain and Privilege: Auto-Ethnographic Collections of Mixed Identity* (Brill, 2019).

Andrew Jakubowicz, Kevin Dunn, Gail Mason, Yin Paradies, Ana-Maria Bliuc, Nasya Bahfen, Andre Oboler, Rosalie Atie, and Karen Connelly, 'Context: 'Cyberspace', 'race' and community resilience', in Andrew Jakubowicz et al., *Cyber Racism and Community Resilience* (Springer, 2017): 1–43.

Jonathan Joseph, 'Resilience as embedded neoliberalism: A governmentality approach', *Resilience* 1/1 (2013): 38–52. https://doi.org/10.1080/21693293.2013.765741

Shahram Khosravi, *'Illegal' Traveller: An Auto-Ethnography of Borders* (Palgrave Macmillan, 2010). https://doi.org/10.1057/9780230281325

Terri Kim, 'Shifting patterns of transnational academic mobility: A comparative and historical approach,' *Comparative Education* (2009), 45(3): 387–403. https://doi.org/10.1080/03050060903184957

Audre Lorde, 'The master's tools will never dismantle the master's house', in *Feminist Postcolonial Theory: A Reader*, edited by Reina Lewis and Sara Mills, (Routledge, 2003): 25–28.

Julie MacLeavy, Maria Fannin, and Wendy Larner, 'Feminism and futurity: Geographies of resistance, resilience and reworking', *Progress in Human Geography* 45/6 (2021). https://doi.org/10.1177/03091325211003327

Nicola Mai, *Mobile Orientations: An Intimate Autoethnography of Migration, Sex Work, and Humanitarian Borders* (University of Chicago Press, 2018).

Mahmood Mamdani, 'Between the public intellectual and the scholar: Decolonization and some post-independence initiatives in African higher education', *Inter-Asia Cultural Studies* 17/1 (2016): 68–83. https://doi.org/10.1080/14649373.2016.1140260

Luca Mavelli, 'Resilience beyond neoliberalism? Mystique of complexity, financial crises, and the reproduction of neoliberal life', *Resilience* 7/3 (2019): 224–239. https://doi.org/10.1080/21693293.2019.1605661

Walter D. Mignolo, 'Delinking', *Cultural Studies* 21/2–3 (2007): 449–514. https://doi.org/10.1080/09502380601162647

Yassir Morsi, *Radical Skin, Moderate Masks: De-Radicalising the Muslim & Racism in Post-Racial Societies* (Rowman & Littlefield Publishers, 2018).

José Esteban Muñoz, 'Ephemera as evidence: Introductory notes to queer acts', *Women and Performance: A Journal of Feminist Theory* 2/8 (1996): 5–12. https://doi.org/10.1080/07407709608571228

PARISS Collective, 'The art of writing social sciences: Disrupting the current politics of style', *Political Anthropological Research on International Social Sciences (PARISS)* 1/1 (2020): 9–38. https://doi.org/10.1163/25903276-bja10008

Larissa Pelúcio, 'Possible appropriations and necessary provocations for a teoria cu' in *Queering Paradigms IV South-North Dialogues on Queer Epistemologies, Embodiments and Activisms*, edited by Sara Elizabeth Lewis, Rodrigo Borba, Branca Falabella, Fabrício de Souza Pinto, and Diana de Souza Pinto (Peter Lang, 2014): 31–52.

Pedro Paulo Gomes Pereira, 'Reflecting on decolonial queer', *GLQ: A Journal of Lesbian and Gay Studies* 25/3 (2019): 403–429.

Ladan Rahbari, 'Peripheral position in social theory: Limitations of social research and dissertation writing in Iran,' *Civitas-Revista de Ciências Sociais* 15 (2015): 155–165. https://doi.org/10.15448/1984-7289.2015.1.18615

Ladan Rahbari, 'Iranian migrant women's shared experiences in Belgium: Where gender, color and religion intersect,' in *The Borders of Integration: Empowered Bodies and Social Cohesion*, edited by Bianca Maria Pirani (Cambridge Scholars, 2018): 203–219.

Ladan Rahbari, 'Recycling my emotions: A 'good' migrant's integration narrative,' *Journal of Narrative Politics* 7/1 (2020): 1–4.

Ladan Rahbari, 'Solidariteit en zelfzorg in neoliberale tijden,' in *Intieme revoluties*, edited by Rahil Roodsaz and Katrien De Graeve (Boom, 2021): 195–208.

Victoria Reyes, *Academic Outsider: Stories of Exclusion and Hope* (Stanford University Press, 2022).

Adrienne Rich, 'Notes toward a politics of location,' in *Women, Feminist Identity and Society in the 1980's: Selected Papers*, edited by Myriam Díaz-Diocaretza and Iris M. Zavala (John Benjamins, 1984): 7–22.

Cecilia L. Ridgeway, 'Why status matters for inequality,' *American Sociological Review* 79/1 (2014): 1–16. https://doi.org/10.1177/0003122413515997

Ralf Roth and Aslı Vatansever, *Scientific Freedom under Attack: Political Oppression, Structural Challenges, and Intellectual Resistance in Modern and Contemporary History* (Campus Verlag, 2020).

Róisín Ryan-Flood and Rosalind Gill, *Secrecy and Silence in the Research Process: Feminist Reflections* (Routledge, 2009).

Katherine J. C. Sang and Thomas Calvard, "I'm a migrant, but I'm the right sort of migrant': Hegemonic masculinity, whiteness, and intersectional privilege and (dis)advantage in migratory academic careers', *Gender, Work & Organization* 26/10 (2019): 1506–1525. https://doi.org/10.1111/gwao.12382

Margrit Shildrick, 'Neoliberalism and embodied precarity: Some crip responses', *South Atlantic Quarterly* 118/3 (2019): 595–613. https://doi.org/10.1215/00382876-7616175

Linda Tuhiwai Smith, *Decolonizing Methodologies: Research and Indigenous Peoples.* (Bloomsbury Publishing, 2021).

Ines Smyth and Caroline Sweetman, 'Introduction: Gender and resilience', *Gender & Development* 23/3 (2015): 405–414. https://doi.org/10.1080/13552074.2015.1113769

Stine H. Bang Svendsen, Kristine Ask, Kristine Øygardslia, Christian Engen Skotnes, Priscilla Ringrose, Gunnar Grut, and Fredrik Røkenes, 'Migration narratives in educational digital storytelling: Which stories can be told?', *Learning, Media and Technology* 47/2 (2021): 201–215. https://doi.org/10.1080/17439884.2021.1954949

Anna Lowenhaupt Tsing, *The Mushroom at the End of the World* (Princeton University Press, 2015).

Eve Tuck and K. Wayne Yang, 'Decolonization is not a metaphor', *Decolonization: Indigeneity, Education & Society* 1/1 (2012): 1–40.

Charikleia Tzanakou & Emily Henderson. 'Stuck and sticky in mobile academia: Reconfiguring the im/mobility binary,' *Higher Education* (2021), 82(4): 685–693. https://doi.org/10.1007/s10734-021-00710-x

Ieva Urbanaviciute, Lara Christina Roll, Jasmina Tomas, and Hans De Witte, 'Proactive strategies for countering the detrimental outcomes of qualitative job insecurity in academia', *Stress and Health* 37/3 (2021): 557–571. https://doi.org/10.1002/smi.3023

Aslı Vatansever, *At the Margins of Academia: Exile, Precariousness, and Subjectivity* (Brill, 2020). https://doi.org/10.1163/9789004431355

Gloria Wekker, *White Innocence* (Duke University Press. 2016).

Andrea Wolvers, 'Introduction', in *Concepts of the Global South*, edited by Andrea Hollington, Tijo Salverda, Tobias Schwarz and Oliver Tappe (Global South Studies Center, 2015).

Michalinos Zembylas, 'The ethics and politics of precarity: Risks and productive possibilities of a critical pedagogy for precarity', *Studies in Philosophy and Education* 38/2 (2019): 95–111. https://doi.org/10.1007/s11217-018-9625-4

Robin Zheng, 'Precarity is a feminist issue: Gender and contingent labor in the academy', *Hypatia* 33/2 (2018): 235–255. https://doi.org/10.1111/hypa.12401

# (NON)BELONGING

# 1. A Journey to the 'Self': From Precarity as Non-Belonging to the Search for Common Ground

*Vera Axyonova*

'It doesn't really matter how smart you are. After we finish our studies, I will be working at a government ministry and you might still end up cleaning floors'. One of my groupmates said this to me during our International Relations course back in my home country. It was meant as a joke. He made it in reference to my belonging to a 'wrong group' and my family's lack of connections which, if existent, would have helped me get a ministerial position. While I did take it as a joke the moment it was told, I couldn't really laugh. The brutal realization that the suggested possibility might (at least to some extent) materialize never escaped my mind. After all, a diploma with honors in International Relations from a provincial university was certainly not a guarantee for a top-notch career, especially without being backed up by the necessary 'add-ons'. A few years later, the same groupmate, who obviously had the right 'add-ons', was indeed working at a ministry, and I found myself in Europe.

I came to Germany in 2006 for my Master's, equipped with a stipend from the German Academic Exchange Service (DAAD) and a great deal of motivation to make the best of the two years ahead of me. A few DAAD stipend holders like myself ended up being in my Master's program—all of us coming from the so-called former Soviet countries, where the DAAD was actively supporting young talent in their pursuit of further education in Germany. As time progressed, I realized we formed a special group within the program, not because

https://doi.org/10.11647/OBP.0331.01

we were all foreigners or because of the 'common communist past' of our home countries, but because our German fellow students saw us as privileged, with DAAD scholarships providing us with a solid financial backing. This was around the time when some German states decided to introduce tuition fees for university students, and many of our course mates complained about their struggles to be able to afford their Master's degrees. The tuition fees did not apply to DAAD scholarship holders. We also received comparably generous funding to support our living and other expenses while in Germany. 'With your stipends you do not have to work to finance your studies like the rest of us', a course mate once told us during a lunch break. 'Well, that is true, but let's wait', my Ukrainian friend replied. 'Once we are done studying, you guys [referring to German students] will be the first to get the good jobs, and we will see about us...'. Turned out she was right.

I was among many foreign students who decided to 'try it' in Germany and one of the very few who quickly found 'something'. In my case, that 'something' was not a job but another... (you guessed it) stipend. A prestigious doctoral stipend for a newly restructured graduate school, in fact. This time, not a support program for foreign students who could 'benefit from studying in the Global North', but a scholarship awarded in an open competition, regardless of the country of origin. Being enormously proud of myself, I felt genuinely privileged, enjoying the intercultural environment of the grad school and intellectually stimulating talks with my peers, the majority of whom were from Germany, other countries in Western Europe, and the US. Yet, the joys of being an international early-career researcher with a full scholarship did not last too long. Outside the university walls, the reality caught up with me quickly at the municipal migration office when the time came to exchange my student visa for a longer-term residence permit.

I remember going to the authoritative (or prison-like) building of the migration office at 5am, hours before it actually opened, during my second attempt to get to the person in charge. My previous attempt was completely in vain, as arriving at the migration office at 9am—when it officially opened—turned out to be much too late to get anywhere beyond the waiting room. With no chance of reaching anyone on the phone or making an appointment online, men and women, some of them with small children and newborns, were standing in front of the migration office's entrance for hours—no matter the weather conditions—just waiting to get inside. Once the security guard opened the doors, the crowd rushed in—literally sprinting up the stairs—to collect the few admission tickets distributed by another security guard for that day. A sign in the doorway over the security guard's head listed the countries and world regions he was responsible for—the whole African continent, Latin America, South and South East Asia, the Western Balkans, and the former Soviet states. A much smaller sign above another doorway listed the US, Canada, Australia, and New Zealand. No one was standing there. I guess the ticket distribution system worked differently for passport holders from those parts of the world.

This was one of many acute moments when I became aware exactly how little the different realities that I was confronted with in my life—as a migrant and as an academic—had in common. Somehow, it reminded me of another incident in the earlier days of my doctoral enrolment. Together with my peers, I was on a train returning from a day-long workshop where we had discussed each other's research projects, many of which focused on fundamental rights, social welfare, precarity, and dividing lines in contemporary societies. While the rigorous discussion still continued on the crowded train, an elderly person passed by, pushing our group apart as he tried to reach for an empty beer bottle standing in the corner. Our group fell silent. 'Wow, that is quite a reality check', one of the fellows said after a while, pointing out how little our talks of precarity and fundamental rights had to do with this person's life and the kind of parallel reality we thought he lived in. Awkwardly though, just a few months later, at the migration office, it was me who felt like living in a parallel reality.

I was struck by how defining such moments seemed to be for my identity and how difficult it was to reconcile my academic 'self' with personal experiences in other spheres of social life. As years passed, I tried to accommodate the different realities I was facing as a scholar and as a person 'with a non-European migration background'. At times, though, I watched these realities clashing as they overlapped across time and space. More than once I asked myself: how do you manage to go to an international conference and give a convincing presentation on the promotion of European values, such as the respect for human dignity, just one day after your own dignity was pretty much kicked in the face at the migration office? Or, how do you explain to a European colleague complaining about the difficulties of traveling to the US 'after the pandemic' that despite following all the rules and being fully vaccinated, there is no chance a person with your color of passport would be granted a visa at the moment? And would you even mention that previously, the effort, time, and money you invested in arranging your conference travel to the UK or the US were by no means comparable to that of the colleague?[1] With your non-European citizenship, you had to spend half a day online just filling out visa application forms, trying to remember which countries you visited in the last ten years (something UK authorities actually ask for) and then another day traveling across the country to the consulate or visa application center for the interview and to submit your files. Finally, how do you react to a German fellow researcher claiming, 'we are all in the same boat, and academic career prospects are equally dim for all young scholars in this country'? How do you explain that you did not have equal chances in German academia at any point in your life? Where do you even start?

Over the years, my initial admiration of the German education and research system, which I aspired to become part of since the start of my Master's studies, was slowly substituted with mild frustration. I realized that, despite the officially promoted appearances of inclusiveness and diversity, the German academic system (and especially the Social Sciences and Humanities domain) remained a privileged club, which did not eagerly open its doors to those coming from outside. There is no need to spend years in the system to understand that, in fact. All it takes is to look at the list of names of political science professors in Germany, prepared by the German Political Science Association in 2017.[2] The proportion of full professors with non-German names is so strikingly low that talking about the internationalization of the country's higher education appears somehow misplaced.

One experience made me realize this more than anything else. Having presented at a large German political science conference, I was

---

1     On inequalities in global academia and access to international conferences see also: Rabe, M., Agboola, C., Kumswa, S., Linonge-Fontebo, H., and Mathe, L. (2021). 'Like a bridge over troubled landscapes: African pathways to doctorateness', *Teaching in Higher Education*, 26/3: 306–320, https://doi.org/10.1080/13562517.2021. 1896490.

2     Politikwissenschaftliche Professuren in Deutschland, www.dvpw.de.

asked by another panelist and a friend of mine if I wanted to join a group of colleagues from his conference section for dinner to celebrate the final day of the event. I gladly agreed, anticipating interesting conversations with peer scholars working on similar issue areas. Although most of the conference was held in English (to attract international participants), we soon switched to German, as discussions developed around the dinner table. This was when it hit me that I was the only non-native speaker in the group. Confident of my fluent German, I tried initiating friendly discussions with a few colleagues sitting next to me. It quickly caught my attention that the only people I could engage with in longer exchanges were the two I knew personally from previous conferences. While others were preoccupied exchanging contact information, deliberating possible cooperation plans, and discussing the current situation on the academic job market, I was somehow not part of any of those conversations. On the way home, I tried to recap the evening in my mind, wondering why that had been the case, until I realized: most of the people at that table may not have seen me as serious competition on the academic market or as someone it would be important to connect with professionally. Considering how very few political science professors at German universities carry a Slavic name, I actually understand why.

There are moments in life that are truly defining, that divide your life into before and after. Such turning points can change the way you see the world and your own 'self'. Many parents would say the day their first child was born was such a moment in their lives; it made them fully reconsider their priorities, both personal and professional. In my case, the moment that changed everything was noon of 1 November 2017, when I saw the last signs of life leaving the little body of my son. After multiple surgeries and almost six months in hospitals and cardiological centers, he could not be saved. Hardly any words can describe the all-devouring pain of loss and of having to live longer than your own child. I will not be searching for those words here—the story of that pain is not for this essay, but the resulting experiences of non-belonging are.

Having survived this major trauma, I made a radical decision to take a break from academic research. I wanted to do something that felt more meaningful than chasing my own dream of becoming a professor. I switched to science management to coordinate a mentoring program for at-risk and displaced scholars, who left their home countries involuntarily, having been pushed out by war, fear of political prosecution, or a humanitarian crisis. Somehow, I associated my personal experiences of trauma with theirs, although our life courses didn't really have much in common. After all, I wasn't forced to leave my country, give up everything I worked for, or be in the limbo of exile. Yet, what I felt connected me with those who had lived through all this was the sense of existential non-belonging, which one acquires through deeply traumatizing experiences.

Non-belonging can take various forms and can be dealt with in different ways. What is common though, is the perception of lacking shared ground with most counterparts in social interactions or groups which one would actually like to be a part of. The sense of non-belonging becomes existential when it is internalized and is not questioned anymore on a daily basis—when it becomes part of one's own identity. It is difficult to avoid for those whose life paths take an extreme turn, such as being abducted and tortured on the way into exile, witnessing the violent deaths of people you know, or losing your children. These are experiences of absolute powerlessness and despair. For those who have never had them, experiences like these are difficult to comprehend and relate to. And for those who have had them, there is no easy way to reconcile them with 'normal' life in a society where crime and death are things you commonly hear about in the news or read in monthly statistics.

Reconciling such experiences with the normality of academic life in apparently meritocracy-driven Global North universities is even more difficult. In a system built on rewarding high-achievers, there is no time and place for those who struggle to recover from trauma, and you are rarely given credit for having managed to do so. Moreover, the ability to adjust is largely taken for granted, excluding those who cannot do that instantly, which only adds further facets to experiencing non-belonging.

Those trying to continue their research work and 'enter' the academic system in their country of exile realize that their new normality is quite different from what they were used to back home. Their previous work and credentials, in many cases, have little value in the new environment. Their publications were all in the 'wrong journals' and in the 'wrong languages', years of teaching experience are depreciated, and their accents give them away as foreigners the minute they start talking.[3]

Academia allows very little space for deviations in what is considered excellent, successful, and trendsetting. As a scientist, you are constantly assessed by your outputs and their quantity and quality (however the latter may be measured). What is never assessed, however, are the personal life circumstances of those behind the outputs, their resilience, and the ability to overcome moments of absolute despair and powerlessness and carry on with the scientific work against all odds.

Working with exiled scholars has shown that to me most bluntly. But it has also taught me that the feeling of non-belonging is fluid and precarity is relative. And both can be mitigated (if not overcome) through experiences of genuine solidarity. In summer 2021, when I closely followed the #ichbinhanna debate on Twitter, I saw it reaffirmed once again. The initiative, started by three younger German scholars to draw public and political attention to the issues of academic precarity, quickly attracted thousands of followers and contributors to the debate. Young and not so young scientists united in their frustration about the university practice of issuing fixed-term contracts for academic positions in Germany and the lack of professional perspectives, preprogrammed by the federal 'legislation exempting university employees from usual labor rights'.[4] Within just a few days, hundreds of academics had shared their very personal stories of precarity, powerlessness, and existential fears. And yes, one could still question whether these stories are in any way comparable when told by a white male scholar with a German passport or by a female scholar of color who is awaiting a decision on her asylum application. And, of course, they are not comparable, and they never will be. But that is also not the only thing I have learned from this initiative. I have learned that solidarity is possible only when you search for common ground, and not for differences.

---

3    Cf. Seyhan, A. (2022). 'Exile in a translational mode: Safeguarding German scholarship in Turkey and the United States during the Nazi reign', in V. Axyonova, F. Kohstall, and C. Richter (eds), *Academics in Exile: Networks, Knowledge Exchange and New Forms of Internationalization*. Transcript.

4    Citation from the English version of the grassroot initiative's website: https://ichbinhanna.wordpress.com/.

Finalizing my work on this essay, I look through all the notes I made in preparation over the last weeks. I realize I could have included many more examples of experiencing precarity as (perceived) powerlessness and non-belonging. However, they would only have reaffirmed what's been said. I decide to draw the line here by sharing one last personal story that has already become my favorite anecdote to laugh about with friends. Having returned to academic work recently, I am looking through literature review articles related to my new research project. As I progress through the texts, I discover that a well-known Central Asian scholar and fellow countryman cites my earlier work in a review of 'Western scholarship' on Central Asia. The irony of it makes me smile. Not only am I cited by someone much more senior and famous in this academic area, but I am also apparently a 'Western scholar', at least in the eyes of a fellow academic from my own country of origin. Regardless of how others see me, what matters more is where I place my 'self'. And if I've learned anything throughout my journey into European academia, it is that the labels others give you by ascribing you to a certain group do not define who you are.

# 2. Unbelonging as a Post-Colonial Predicament: My Tryst With European Academia

*Sanam Roohi*

I am an accidental academic. Don't get me wrong, I do not suffer from any severe form of imposter syndrome (Wilkinson, 2020) and have enjoyed learning and teaching from a very young age. In fact, I think teaching is my *ikigai* (reason for being). As the second eldest in a large family of six siblings and four cousins, it was my default task to teach my younger siblings and cousins, and even neighbors. The most fulfilling part of my academic life so far was when I slogged as an assistant professor at a university in Bangalore, doing 18 hours of contact teaching with Bachelor's and Master's students every week. I use the term 'teaching' here in a rather uncomplicated way, fully aware that it is not a top-down process and is co-created between students and teachers. So, when I say I am an accidental academic, I mean I never planned or foresaw myself becoming a part of the community of scholars who engage in intellectual debate and knowledge production, not till I left my first job after my Master's. Yet today, with a PhD degree from the University of Amsterdam and having worked in German academia for more than four years, I have become a part of the growing group of migrant academics in Europe whose relationship with academia is often tenuous—threatened by an end date when the fellowship concludes and the visa expires. In this short piece, I reflect upon the struggles and embodied negotiations I experience as a temporary job-holder who is a part of the growing 'international academic precariat' (Drążkiewicz, 2021).

    https://doi.org/10.11647/OBP.0331.02

## Learning through trial and error

I am a first-generation university graduate and my academic journey so far has been about learning and adapting through trial and error. With no experience within my (extended) family to fall back upon, I have always found academia to be both alienating and emancipatory. That contradictory feeling persists to this date. While my corporeal marking in India as that of a Muslim girl always threatened to 'other' me and make me a misfit in my classroom ('Muslim girls are not interested in studies', 'they are married off early', 'they are forced to wear *burkha*' were some familiar refrains I'd hear in school), because of my current physical location in the Western part of the globe, I am marked as a brown body—inherent within whom is the valued currency of diversity but the use of which is only temporary and marginal. Traversing through India and Europe, there are many overt and covert ways in which both these markers have inflected my precarious academic life.

Notwithstanding the precarity, I owe it to my mother and aunt who laid the foundations of my academic journey. In my world, they are the giants on whose shoulders I've stood, rather than being guided by any academic mentor, the repercussions of which are hard to miss. It was my aunt who dreamed of an *English medium*1 education for us, marching up to school after school and learning the ropes of getting the coveted 'admission'. She set the ball of aspiration rolling but got married soon after, and the task of our schooling fell on our 'uneducated' mother who had only studied till the fourth standard because the middle school was in a neighboring village and girls from conservative Muslim families did not have a lot of freedom to travel for education in rural India in the late 1960s. Married to my father in a big metropolitan city, she was enamored by educated women, the respect they commanded and the financial independence some of them had. She regretted her own lack of formal education and told us sisters repeatedly 'you all must at least be a graduate and stand on your own feet. You should become (school) teachers...it brings you respect'. I agreed with only the first half of this advice and went on to do an Honors degree in political science with the aim of becoming a

---

1    While ubiquitous now, English medium education is associated with India's growing middle class and their global aspirations (see Sancho, 2016 for details).

journalist or working in some think-tank—inspired as I was with the discipline of international relations. My love for the discipline did not last long once I got into the MA program.

I discovered my (in hindsight, not unproblematic) adoration for academia during my Master's. My professors, aloof and distant yet scholarly, opened my intellectual vista to the possibilities of knowledge, introducing me to the thoughts of Marx and Gandhi, Arendt and Foucault, Said and Chatterjee among many others. I thought knowledge for knowledge's sake was a noble pursuit beyond an instrumentalist end to enter the job market. I did get a job right after my Master's, working in a small research institute for 18 months, which introduced me to the whole environment that makes up higher education and research. While my work was largely administrative, I realized that I wanted to be a part of a coveted circle of erudite men and women who got together for workshops and conferences, and shared (but mostly exhibited) their knowledge. I set a self-goal to get into a PhD program and picked migration as my topic of interest. But beyond these two vague objectives, my plans were unclear. In the face of resistance, I also moved cities to marry a man who belonged to a different caste, religion, and region—an increasingly difficult proposition in a rapidly radicalizing India.

Indian academia overwhelmingly consists of people belonging to the upper castes who have (often unreflexively) set the higher education and research agenda circumscribed by their own caste and class locations. The last couple of decades has seen many first-generation graduates from marginalized communities challenging their hegemony. Yet, outside of the classed, casted, and deeply privileged Indian academic circles, PhD horror stories circulate regularly. Relations between students and their supervisors are described as feudalistic and extractive—the worst of which entails all forms of abuse, and the better of which entails a perpetual relation of subservience. This was a key reason, apart from the coveted international degree and shrinking academic freedom, why I planned to study abroad. The US was my desired PhD destination, but without enough resources to prepare for the GRE exam and being unsure of myself, I chanced upon a PhD project that suited me just fine—a collaborative PhD program (Bourdeau et al., 2007; Banks and Bhandari, 2012; Knight, 2012; Almieda et Al., 2019), for which I had to be in India most of the time with short travels to the Netherlands, and would be awarded a degree from the University of Amsterdam if I successfully defended my thesis. Touted as an ideal blend of providing international training to 'developing' countries' students without necessarily fostering their migration to the 'developed' world for a degree, inequality and an anti-migration agenda is inherent in these programs (as I was about to experience for myself).

## PhDs—*Rites de passage* or cheap (racialized) laboring bodies?

The start of my PhD marked my real entrance into academia. In the absence of any credible networks to rely on, I navigated my fledging academic aspirations by the simple diktat: just keep moving forward, one step at a time. What I did not take into account in this simplistic, almost algorithmic logic was the messiness of human emotions and the power relations that can make or break academic careers. It took me six years to complete my PhD and get a degree and these six (in my perception, long) years brought me into close contact with the realities that many have experienced in their academic trajectory but only a few have written about. Like any other structure designed to ensure that the balance of power resides with the powerful, academia too rewards those with position and rank who accrue more power in the process. The gendered reproduction in academia and the disciplinary limitations on women and people of color has garnered some scholarly attention (Muhs et Al., 2012; Behl, 2019). Certain institutions have also come under intense scrutiny[2] more than others. But perhaps what has not been discussed much is how the PhD has transformed from a rite of passage to enter academia under a mentor's tutelage to becoming a way for group leaders and principal investigators to have access to cheap but skilled labor to gather primary data in labs and fields, with no commitment to long-term mentorship.

---

2    Vita Peacock's work (2016) on the Max Planck Society (MPS) highlights how the Dumontian paramount values of excellence engender hierarchy and dependence, where the directors with a permanent position encompass their subordinates, who have contractual jobs. It generated a lot of discussions thereafter, which were published in the journal HAU as rejoinders, including those of Julie Billaud and Cristoph Brumann.

As part of a couple of Facebook groups where doctoral and post-doctoral researchers share their academic experiences, anxieties, and problems, I have read many entries that tackle issues of gendered or racial discrimination, but exploitation is still rarely discussed—either out of fear or the feeling that it is the natural order of things, 'part of the bargain'. A few posts or memes that do hint about this under-represented aspect of academic practice receive huge responses in the forms of likes, perhaps exhibiting silent solidarity or even identification with the author's travail. Of course, PhD supervision and mentorship are relations of dependence where power is always skewed. But in such protracted and often intense interpersonal dynamics, there is a fine line that distinguishes subordination and subjugation from enabling forms of stewardship.

My PhD was part of a program designed to have two India-based students who would visit Amsterdam twice for three months during their four-year project and one Netherlands-based PhD student who would have the opposite arrangement, with the final defense of our thesis at the University of Amsterdam. Because of the collaborative nature of the PhD, I had to fulfil the academic obligations of two institutes—one in India and the other in the Netherlands—while being paid one-sixth of my Dutch counterpart. Given my work on migration, the parallels of my situation with the literature critiquing migration management and the governance practices that expect migrants to be temporary (thus paving the way for their return to the home country and preventing their integration in the host country) were not lost on me. In case we missed the implications, we were repeatedly reminded by our Dutch colleague that we should stay in our country after the degree and not look for jobs in the Western part of the globe! Apart from the structural biases, discrimination in supervision, the hierarchization of team members based on their skin color, online surveillance (keeping a tab of what we posted on our social media), encounters with forms of casual racism (not just offensive stereotyping but opinions held on such prejudices) was part of the package. But more than the blatant forms of discrimination inscribed in the design of the PhD program—including gross underpayment, bias in supervision, or more than double the workload (including administrative work and work without any stipend in the fifth year of the PhD)—it was the lack of any institutional recourse generally available to other students who were fully immersed in either of the institutes that left me most vulnerable. After working remotely, the second India-based PhD colleague eventually and unsurprisingly dropped out of the program.

Within the first year of the PhD, I completed the compulsory coursework, acquired the required credits (receiving As in all the graded courses), cleared the comprehensive exam, and had my eight-month paper—a 40-plus page review paper-cum-proposal submitted to a committee in the department—positively evaluated. The toughest phase, however, began thereafter, when I left for the year-long fieldwork. I realized that, behind the trappings of a PhD degree from a world-renowned university and the promise to have my own autonomous project, I was ultimately a research assistant, whose job was primarily to collect data and field insights for the supervisors. At one point halfway through the fieldwork, as I simultaneously wrote a 40-page field report, prepared for my supervisors' weeklong visit to my fieldsite, organized a half-day workshop with my respondents, and simultaneously prepared for the US leg of fieldwork (visa, tickets, accommodation, contacts etc., without any institutional help), I fell behind in typing my daily notes. My India-based supervisor punished me by making me cancel my US field trip, ultimately allowing me to reschedule my trip to a month later, after I had finished typing all the notes. Other arbitrary rules were set, forbidding me from attending conferences or working on publications other than the monograph—rules that were not applied to my Dutch teammate.

After an Indian post-doc was unceremoniously ousted from the program in the first year, I was gripped by a constant fear that I was replaceable, and if ousted, I would be alienated from my work that I felt passionate about—a fear that I feel, in hindsight, was recognized by my supervisors, who weaponized it against me. A supervisor even pointed out during my defense that I'd never broken down or called it quits! Finishing the degree became my solitary goal and by the end of the fourth year, I had submitted my work-in-progress monograph for feedback. The only feedback I did receive was being asked to rewrite my thesis completely from scratch because the present thesis 'dealt with too many things'. The decision felt not only arbitrary but unjust, because previous chapter submissions had received no feedback from one supervisor, while the other always gave me encouraging verbal feedback. After the cool dismissal of the thesis without any proper explanation, the memory of being forced to join the group dinner that evening evokes a deeply unsettling feeling even today. Determined not to let this development break me, I started writing my thesis from scratch the very next day and submitted a second draft a year later. Unfortunately, my Dutch supervisor passed away before he could read the new thesis. It was only when a new supervisor came on board that I realized the significance of professionalism in a field that openly exhibits its reliance on networks and patronage as a badge of honor. Thanks to the new supervisor's swift feedback and interjections, I submitted my thesis to the committee a few months after he took over, and successfully defended my thesis at the University of Amsterdam.

After the thesis submission, I decided to take up a teaching job I was offered in a Bangalore college, which many in India consider to be a professional downgrade for international PhD students. After much deliberation, I also decided to make a clean break from the toxic professional relations I had to endure during my PhD, which still had me in their grip—a decision which would have far-reaching repercussions. I did not take this decision in haste but after careful consideration, fully aware that much of my academic prospects in India—and some abroad— would be over in the process. While consumed by teaching six days a week, I decided that giving up on research was not worth the travails I had endured earlier. I started working on a couple of publications and took unpaid leave for self-funded fieldwork trips, experimenting with a few vastly different research ideas. Twenty months into the teaching job, when I least expected it, I received a Marie Curie COFUND fellowship in Germany, and I made the tough decision to resign from my teaching job and move to Germany in search of a fulfilling academic career.

## Unbelonging as a (post-)colonial predicament

After Said, many scholars working on/in the East have written extensively about the post-colonial predicament the post-colonies and their inhabitants have to contend with (Breckenridge and van der Veer, 1993). As mobile academics from the Global South, our predicaments are compounded by our knowledge of the epistemic foundations of our scholarly encounters and adventures. As reflexive beings, we not only carry forward identities and categories inherited from our colonial past: they are made and remade dialectically, co-constituted by our subjective experiences and interactions within the international academic setting. Even as our mobility privileges us in many ways, our post-colonial predicament presents itself in myriad other ways that may not offset the privilege but often reduce us to our national, racial, or ethnic identities.

Working for more than four years in German academia as a post-doc in two different institutes on two different fellowships, for the first time I've felt like my work is valued and my autonomy has been regained. I sometimes marvel at my luck at being paid to read and write (and teach, though not obligatorily). At a time when many countries across the globe see social sciences as redundant, it is heartening to see Germany not only provide financial and infrastructural support for quality social science research, but also give ample space to researchers to do their work without much institutional interference (and despite the bureaucratic hurdles). While in Germany the prospects for funding are high and the infrastructure is mostly top quality, not everyone succeeds in securing funding, flexibility (read: job insecurity) is encouraged, and universities do not support researchers beyond six years. The lack of tenure has prompted the #ichbinhanna movement (where accomplished post-docs and adjuncts exposed the system that encourages insecurity in the name of flexibility) to trend on Twitter in May and June 2021.[3]

My predicament is shown most starkly in this situation. I fully support the cause but I did not feel comfortable enough to join it, lest I be considered an interloper. After all, I am an outsider who does not even speak German (fully, yet) and is just a temporary researcher in Germany. During my PhD I was constantly reminded that I was an offshore worker, and as a post-doc, I feel more akin to a guestworker who is expected to do the stipulated task and leave. In fact, my situation is not very different from that of guestworkers of yesteryear, with one noteworthy difference—their contribution was significant in the rebuilding of post-war Germany, while my contributions are often meant for the limited consumption of a small academic circle. And even

---

3    In the last couple of months, the #ichbinhanna movement has trended on Twitter protesting the normalization of job insecurity and flexibility in German academia, https://www.timeshighereducation.com/news/ichbinhanna-german-researchers-snap-over-lack-permanent-jobs

as I plan to stay here and build a career, I may not be successful, and if I do succeed, the journey will certainly not be easy.

The reification of the nation and national belonging is not limited to ordinary Germans, but is rife in academia too. Perhaps unlike US academia, the idea of (academic) positions 'in Germany for Germans' is an unspoken rule that many outsiders have to contend with. Some German academics I meet take it for granted that my time in Germany is limited and expect me to return to my country (to which I feel increasingly alienated from). Having spoken to a few of my fellow non-European colleagues about our particular kind of precarity (unlike other EU citizens, we do not have the privilege of staying even a day longer than our contract or stipend[4] lasts and our visa expires), they reveal similar anxieties. There seems to be a hierarchy in Germany where permanent academic positions are (perhaps based on some precept of *naturalness*) reserved for its citizens. As foreigners, you may stay on, as long as you succeed in getting funded for your temporary positions. I have applied to a couple of tenure track positions in Germany and got called for an interview for one of them. A professor whom I reached out for advice hinted that I should not get up my hopes, because the competition for these severely limited positions is extremely high, knowing German is a prerequisite and jobs are secured through 'networks'. During difficult times, I am reminded of a meeting I had with one Indian researcher at a Max Planck Institute (who had many excellent publications and academic feats under her belt) telling me quite tersely that I should not dream of making an academic career in Germany. Giving her own example, she exclaimed: 'I feel like a beggar, surviving from project to project and perpetually writing applications. I have a reason to stay here (marriage to a German) but you should not. Rather aim for the US'.

The anxieties surrounding my temporary situation impinge not only on my academic productivity, but also on the relationships I build.

---

4    Contractual job holders can avail the Blue Card program that allows qualified academics to stay in Germany for three years, but early versions of it came with restrictions of language and salary limits. As of 2023, rules have been modified to allow for greater ease of mobility for non-EU members to stay in Germany but the conditions of a job contract with a salary threshold (58,000 Euros in non-STEM fields) still remains. As for academics who receive a stipend, the rule of returning to their country of origin the day their visa expires is still in place, disproportionately affecting many non-EU fellowship holders.

During the first year of my stay in Germany, I invited every member of my cohort and a few others for dinners, and it remained mostly unreciprocated. In my more than a decade of association, I am still surprised by many Europeans' inability to share meals. That does not stop them from inviting themselves over for 'curry' dinners, however! In such an equal setting, friendships become fleeting and temporary; forging meaningful relationships becomes difficult.

In Germany, the East/West divide and the language barrier are additional problems one has to deal with. My first fellowship (initially for a year, but extended to another after I successfully won another round) was in an institute which I personally feel has been the best place I have worked in so far. But my experience with the city was quite the opposite. As an East German town, it is known to be unkind to foreigners, and every brown/black body is seen as an unwelcome refugee. Barely a few days after moving to the city, at the city registration office I was scolded for not knowing German. The scolding turned grisly at the tax office. The language barrier felt insurmountable with the increasing number of interactions I had with native speakers. I decided to learn German, but courses clashed with my fieldwork initially and with no knowledge of whether I would be in the country for longer, I deferred learning the language professionally till I moved to another city for my second fellowship. I find German a difficult language to learn, and after ten months of evening classes twice a week, I still have a long way to go. In fact, the fear of not speaking the language is so paralyzing that I (and some others I know) avoid going to the doctor or seeking any other kind of professional help as long as we can.

Living in Germany during the pandemic also brought home the realization that the chasm between the Global North and South is not just about the economy or the market, or even the healthcare system. The differences are embodied and affective. During India's first wave of COVID-19, I spent hours talking to my extended family, childhood friends, and neighbors, explaining to them whatever little knowledge I had of the virus—teaching them caution and perhaps assuaging my guilt of staying in a relatively safer place through it. The virus still wreaked havoc in my family, killing my beloved uncle who loved me dearly. Not being there for him and not being able to say goodbye guts me, even two years after his passing. The fact that one can have strong bonds with relatives who are not one's parents or grandparents is perhaps outside of the grasp of many Europeans, who could not sympathize with my loss. But the fear I felt in the first wave multiplied manifold with the second wave; I had constant prayers on my lips, eyes glued to news channels and social media for two months straight. Amplifying the calls for help and donating to volunteers via social media platforms became my way of reaching out from afar. And as some of us from the Global South suffered, the lack of empathy around us was initially shocking, till I realized that Europeans (particularly Germans) were largely shielded by their proactive government actions and superior healthcare systems, and empathy can only be built if one either goes through or witnesses devastation first hand.

## Parting thoughts

Despite the gnawing and ever-present precarity I am in, after spending more than a decade in academia, I (perhaps like many in my situation), do not wish to change my vocation. At times, I also feel ill-equipped to survive outside of academia, but it does not deter me from imagining alternate lives I could have led. These imaginary alternatives appear tantalizing, with the promise of a stable job, steady income, and work-life balance. I also reminisce about the fateful day—18 February 2010—when I had started from home in an autorickshaw to go for the PhD interview. Halfway through, I got a call from the manager at Nokia, Bangalore office, with a job offer. During the interview held a few months earlier, she had ominously narrated how she had switched from academia to the corporate sector, thoroughly disillusioned with the former. When she called back with an offer, I did not hesitate to decline it immediately, despite not knowing what the outcome of the interview would be, because I strongly felt that academia was my true calling. Today, if I ever begin to question my choice, I immediately recollect what academia has given me so far—the possibility to pursue my passion for research and teaching—and the feeling dissipates in seconds. And even if I may not feel I wholly belong here, my love for research and teaching belongs to me.

# Works cited

Joana Almeida, Sue Robson, Marilia Morosini, and Caroline Baranzeli, 'Understanding internationalization at home: Perspectives from the global North and South,' *European Educational Research Journal* 18/2 (2019): 200–217. https://doi.org/10.1177/1474904118807537

Melissa Banks and Rajika Bhandari, 'Global student mobility,' *The SAGE Handbook of International Higher Education* (2012): 379–397.

Natasha Behl, 'Mapping movements and motivations: An autoethnographic analysis of racial, gendered, and epistemic violence in academia', *Feminist Formations*, 31/1 (2019): 85–102. https://doi.org/10.1353/ff.2019.0010

Julie Billaud, 'No wonder! Kingship and the everyday at the Max Planck Society', *HAU: Journal of Ethnographic Theory*, 6/1 (2016): 121–126. https://doi.org/10.14318/hau6.1.007

Jacqueline Bourdeau, France Henri, Aude Dufresne, Josephine Tchetagni, and Racha Ben Ali, 'Collaborative learning and research training: Towards a doctoral training environment,' *Les Cahiers Leibniz: Laboratoire Leibniz-IMAG, Grenoble, France*, 157 (2007): 38–47.

Carol A. Breckenridge and Peter van der Veer (eds), *Orientalism and the Postcolonial Predicament: Perspectives on South Asia* (Philadelphia: University of Pennsylvania Press, 1993).

Christoph Brumann, 'Max Planck dependence, in context', *HAU: Journal of Ethnographic Theory*, 6/1 (2016): 131–134. https://doi.org/10.14318/hau6.1.009

Ela Drążkiewicz, '*Blinded by the Light: International Precariat in Academia*' (2021), https://www.focaalblog.com/2021/02/05/ela-drazkiewicz-blinded-by-the-light-international-precariat-in-academia/.

Jane Knight, 'Student mobility and internationalization: Trends and tribulations', *Research in Comparative and International Education*, 7/1 (2012): 20–33. http://dx.doi.org/10.2304/rcie.2012.7.1.20

Gabriella Gutiérrez y Muhs, Yolanda Flores Niemann, Carmen G. Gonzalez, and Angela P. Harris (eds), *Presumed Incompetent: The Intersections of Race and Class For Women in Academia* (Utah State University Press, 2012).

Vita Peacock, 'Academic precarity as hierarchical dependence in the Max Planck Society', *HAU: Journal of Ethnographic Theory*, 6/1 (2016): 95–119. https://doi.org/10.14318/hau6.1.006

David Sancho, 'Keeping up with the time': Rebranding education and class formation in globalising India', *Globalisation, Societies and Education*, 14/4/ (2016): 477–491. https://doi.org/10.1080/14767724.2015.1077101

Catherine Wilkinson, 'Imposter syndrome and the accidental academic: An autoethnographic account', *International Journal for Academic Development*, 25/4 (2020): 363–374. https://doi.org/10.1080/1360144X.2020.1762087

# 3. Unlearning

## *Mihnea Tănăsescu*

I left home when I was 16. At the time, home was Bucharest, Romania. I'd be lying if I said that I had any trouble leaving—I was ready and willing. True, I loved the summer rain storms and the specific sense of humor of the place, but I was also choked by the aggressiveness of a society unravelling in a contradictory vise: one side totalitarian, the other capitalist consumerist. I wanted to leave. Today, most of my friends from that period no longer live in the country of their birth. Mine was a shared feeling.

Looking back, I was a child when I left. Then, it felt like I had already lived a lifetime, and was ready for another one. What I didn't know, couldn't know, was the vastness of the world and the tantalizing possibility of belonging to many places, many people, many ways of knowing. I also didn't know that this possibility would be both a benefit and a drawback. I did not know that, after learning so much, I would have to unlearn as well.

My first adoptive home was Italy. I had received a scholarship to attend the United World College of the Adriatic for the last two years of high school—an international school dedicated to building peace through education. I almost didn't make it there, because the visa officer at the Italian consulate refused to issue a visa. Following my mom's lead, we simply changed tellers and found a public servant that was willing to issue a visa. My whole trajectory of being an authorized migrant started with a bureaucratic happenstance.

My second adoptive country was the United States, where I spent seven years studying and doing odd jobs to survive (I learned at least as much from these as from formal schooling). After that period, I decided to move yet again, this time to Belgium, where my sister had a

 https://doi.org/10.11647/OBP.0331.03

free couch that I could sleep on. Because Romania had recently joined the European Union, this was the first time that I had traveled without advanced planning that required humiliating prostrations before consulate officials that held my fate in their hands. After years of having to periodically reauthorize my status as a migrant (an 'alien' in the US), I had become a 'European citizen'. Personally, it was a welcome change, as it would allow frictionless travel—a tremendous luxury. More generally, it exposed the facade of equal treatment; nothing at all had changed in who I was or what I did, and yet I was now free to go unquestioned to where I couldn't go before without very lengthy questioning.

Moving to Belgium meant restarting everything again: learning new languages, making new friends, finding a new job. I didn't mind any of it. By chance, I found a PhD position in political science (a subject I had never studied before) and began, without knowing it, my 'career' in academia. I settled in Brussels, where I have lived ever since. Twelve years later, I am writing these words as an eternal post-doc pushing 40.

My time 'away from my country' has come to seem like a contradictory experience of acceptance and rejection. This is not a strictly personal experience; it seems to be common among people with a 'migrant background'. Paradoxically, I never really thought of myself as a migrant because I had always been privileged enough to penetrate the unmarked centers of power that allowed me to live a decent life. My privilege didn't come from wealth or status, but from youth and skin color: I was a voluble white man, and this allowed me to slip through spaces that may have been much tighter had I been perceived as more exotic.

Mind you, I *was* exotic for many people. In the United States, for example, people routinely had no idea where Romania was, or what Romanian sounded like, and were generally very interested in me, in the way of a museum exhibit that enlivens the day and gives a jolt of momentary excitement. I benefited from this position that I couldn't but inhabit, a ledge between being not exotic enough, and being too much so. I had very little to do with the history of racism and classism in the US and could therefore afford to be safely detached from the violence that that history generates. I was therefore white and not white at the same time, and that worked, for a while. In other words, I used my exoticism for my own benefit, and I have no doubt that part of the reason

I received a US scholarship in the first place was for my catalogue value as an asset to diversity.

In Italy and Belgium, the experience of being 'other' also existed, but in completely different ways. Because of the stigma that had accompanied Romanian migrations since the beginning of the 1990s, people were routinely surprised that I was Romanian, that I was camouflaged so well. I cannot count the number of times I heard that I don't *seem* Romanian, which was always said as a kind of compliment, as if my perceived distance from my stereotypical co-nationals was a badge of honor. I never knowingly distanced myself from a 'Romanian identity', but in fact reveled in the contradictions that my nationality provoked.

This meant that I never lost an opportunity to state my origins. It helps that I have had many such opportunities, because people routinely asked me where I was from, a question that became less and less intelligible the more I switched and traveled and learned. But I always said 'I'm Romanian', precisely because I knew that most of the time the—'but you don't seem Romanian'—would follow, even if not actually said. I always naïvely hoped that people would realize the absurdity of that statement, and perhaps unlearn the habits of mind that led to it.

It took me a long time to realize that I also continued being *too Romanian*. In academia, the latest fashion is for outward acceptance of diversity. Paradoxically, this has reinforced the notion that a person has a primary identity, either white, or black, or queer, or what have you. Of course, everyone is free to identify as they wish. But what often escapes the consideration of the most educated of society is that a person may be multiple things, at once.

There are several ways of illustrating this. Let's start with language: in Dutch, there is a famous (and infamous) distinction between allochthon and autochthon. The latter means a true local, one that traces their genealogy back an unspecified amount of time, but especially one that can be unproblematically counted as a member of the Dutch-speaking community, given outwardly visible traits. An allochthon, on the other hand, is someone of dubious belonging, not because of birth (this term is routinely applied to third generation citizens), but because they may harbor multiple belongings. Usually, this is indicated by outward signs, like looking different.

In my case, being able to pass as white in the general definition that the West has constructed, the allochthon status is confirmed by the origin question: where are you from? This ties my being to my place of birth, even though I have become multiple, multiple times over. I have traces of and allegiances to many places, reflected through the languages I speak and the abiding interest in the environments that hosted me and have become home. Being tied to a place of birth in effect denies the multiplicity of the person; it corrals the many-dimensional person into a stereotype.

This happens in academia as much as elsewhere, but it is mostly unacknowledged and, many times, unconscious. Let's illustrate it another way. As an academic, you are expected to belong to a discipline. Universities are busy outdoing each other in proclaiming their commitment to interdisciplinarity, though in my experience having multiple roots in multiple ways of seeing and thinking is a definite career drawback. You become unplaceable, just as someone with no place of birth: you cannot be from nowhere! If you are academically multiple, and therefore from nowhere, you become a museum exhibit once again, someone that looks good on the catalogue but whose ability to teach Political Science 101 is constantly doubted and practically denied.

Because of the disciplinary and conservative structure of most academic institutions, interdisciplinary scholars are forced to apply for positions in departments run by monodisciplinary people. In my academic background, I have studied human ecology, philosophy, and political science, and have done recognized work in all these fields plus environmental social science, critical jurisprudence, and human geography. I routinely draw on ecology, biology, and cartography. Perhaps my tolerance for academic multiplicity is tied to my tolerance for the cultural kind, I don't know. What I do know is that these professional abilities, supposedly sought after by everyone, quickly become a drawback when, for example, I apply for a job in a sociology department. Or a human geography one. Or political science. Judged on the merits of the discipline itself, I will never be able to compete with traditional careers.

It is as if one must have the courage to be interdisciplinary. I hate that word, 'interdisciplinary'; it means nothing since it has become a marketing ploy. What I mean is that scholars that are passionate about *problems,* and therefore reach wherever necessary to understand them, need more time to learn all of the different salient points of view; their work will take longer to publish because most journal and book reviewers are not versed in multiple disciplines; and they will therefore have to take the risks associated with a career choice that is ostensibly supported but practically not.

More and more young scholars are multiple in their belonging, but must function within institutions that, at least subliminally, want them to conform to a pre-given idea. I suspect that, to most autochthons in Flemish academia, where I currently work, there would rarely be someone *partly* Flemish. To be clear: the academic environment I know is politically progressive and consistently critical of nativist discourse. In practice, however, the institution itself requires a level of belonging to the Flemish identity (itself constructed, of course) that de facto excludes multiplicity. You can be from Antwerp and live in Brussels (though even that is a stretch!), but it is hard to imagine that one may feel just as home in Italy, Romania, the United States, and Belgium. The multiple feeling of home is an unadulterated good. It is also an untapped asset for academic institutions that fail to recognize it as such.

A last illustration of the persistent denial of multiplicity: academics are indoctrinated in a toxic publishing culture that demands constant quantity. This is summed up by the famous (at least in academic circles) saying, 'publish or perish'. There is a strict hierarchy of what counts as worthy publications as well, and every academic in the social sciences must go through the process of learning this unstated order of things. Articles are more valuable than books, edited volumes less valuable than monographs (single-authored books), and so on. At the same time, the venue of publication is also implicitly ranked, feeding into a predatory publication industry that thrives on academic dogmatism and insecurity. Being multiple in your publication choices is not a smart career move.

Functioning within a hyper-competitive environment that requires allegiance through conformity to a set of practices (e.g. constantly publishing your work) is a kind of education. As I have progressed in my career, though all of it was precarious from a contractual point of view, I too have internalized the norms of uniformity that go against my multiple belongings, as well as my moral compass. By any reasonable measure, I have published too much; by current academic standards, I have published too little. I have also internalized the ranking of form and venue, and have routinely lost more time on meeting those standards than on developing the ideas themselves.

Ostensibly, I am all about ethical publishing, slow science, open access, and so on. Practically, I have done very little to live by those principles. And so, last year, as I was contemplating unemployment (and eventually experiencing it for the first time), the whole cycle of temporary contract—application—rejection—application—publication—publication—application—end—restart had gotten a bit too much. I realized that I couldn't go on living by those standards when I noticed that, upon receiving good news, I felt no joy. This was a devastating observation. After all, joy is one of those feelings that punctuates life in a way that outlives its momentary nature; without joy, what else is there? My gradual education in monotony had imperiled this life-giving feeling.

That observation imposed a distance between what I had learned I had to do to be an academic, and what I wanted to continue doing. This opened up the space for unlearning, painful and slow and anything but linear. It started with accepting unemployment benefits—thankfully available in Belgium—as the well-earned social safety net that generations of labor struggles had secured. It was admittedly hard to get there, but it eventually worked. Instead of writing the same article yet another time, I saw that this was the ideal time to write those books that had been brewing within, but never had the space to come out. Career-wise, in my disciplinary circles, not a good move; it would have made more 'sense' to break the ideas up into articles, which in political science, for example, are counted as more important than books.

Regardless, I wrote. For the first time in my academic life, I wrote like I wanted to, without compromises on form or content. It all came pouring out, in what could be called a joyful process.

Then came another really hard part of unlearning: where do I choose to publish? I had been trained for years to think that University Presses are superior to Commercial Publishers that are superior to Open Access publishers committed to changing the publication system altogether. I instinctively followed this model, though I knew all too well how untenable and unfair and frankly ridiculous it was. It is well known that University Presses often prefer insiders over outsides, and that Commercial Publishers are little more than multinational conglomerates skimming off public research money to make a hefty profit. Most academics know this, but most academics have also internalized a hierarchical, uniform structure that keeps the prestige of certain presses intact.

Within the various categories of publishers, there is also an internal hierarchy. For example, in the for-profit commercial camp, there is a clear preference for the largest conglomerates, which a Google search would suffice to reveal (for non-academics, as academics know them all too well). Deciding that, given my precarious status, I did not want to write my manuscripts without knowing that they would be published, I approached the usual suspects that my miseducation had inculcated. I was offered a contract by one big corporate player and accepted it. Admittedly, I barely read the contract. My training rendered that unnecessary; I had made it.

I then spent months writing. Eventually, I had a draft, the best work I had ever done, born out of passion and the gradual unlearning of dependency on acceptance. A new post-doc contract unexpectedly made things financially better, which further freed me to write as I pleased. I sent the draft to the publisher. Their quick response, though positive—they liked it—also made me realize that they hadn't really read it. Commercial presses of this size live on quantity and unpaid labor, so of course they didn't carefully read it! I also realized that my book was going to be placed in a series that had nothing to do with it, and that it would cost 120 UK pounds.

This is very familiar to anyone that has published an academic book, and regrettably common practice. In many different discussions with peers, we complained about this model and the exorbitant prices charged for books that the public had already paid for. I therefore wrote to my editor to ask if the series could be changed, and if they would consider simultaneously releasing a paperback edition at a reasonable price. They declined, over and over again. Their bottom line was that they needed to sell X number of copies to libraries, and putting out a paperback would of course make the expensive version unattractive.

This bottom-line thinking makes no sense from an author's point of view. I am not in it to sell to a hundred libraries and line the pockets of predatory publishers. Given the fundamental disagreement between us, I started contemplating terminating the contract. After (finally) carefully reading it, I learned that there was no way for me as an author to terminate it; only the publisher had this right. So, I got in touch with my editor and, citing irreconcilable differences, I asked to be released. Half an hour later, they let me go, no questions asked.

I felt liberated and confused. Did they care this little about me? Was it really nothing else than a business transaction? My own naïveté was shocking; what was I thinking? Hadn't it always been clear that these publishers don't give a shit? It had, but... Really?

Really. And so, I plunged into looking for another publisher. At first, I wrote to one at a time, waiting for weeks for a reply. Graduating from this alienating experience, I wrote to many at once, waiting for replies that mostly never arrived, or getting immediate rejections with no feedback. Throughout this process, I had my eye on several Open Access Presses with explicit political agendas and transparent, ethical standards. I knew their work and knew that they published books that were at least as good as what more prestigious presses published. They also took risks, accepted truly interdisciplinary work, and had things like explicit anti-slavery policies and a commitment to acknowledging authors and moving the review and publication process along briskly. Because these presses are not for profit, they don't have a quantity target per year, and so they publish whatever they see as good work (always rigorously peer-reviewed) on a rolling basis. This makes so much sense. But I still couldn't get myself to submit my manuscript to them, fearing it deep inside. I thought that I wasn't yet in a position to choose the publisher that had the best practices, because I still needed to prove myself (seven years after my PhD! That's precarity for you). Academic forums and threads confirmed that the publisher matters, that if your book is not with a 'top' press, nobody will consider it worthy.

Given the price that my initial publisher would have charged people for my work, I intuited that it just could not be that having the book in open access would have it travel *less*. If nothing else, I would have been ashamed to promote a book that cost that much, even if it was mine. And yet I couldn't submit to Open Access Publishers. The unlearning was ongoing; I wasn't far enough.

Eventually, I grew so exhausted of the long-established publication model that I sent it to an Open Access Publisher. To my complete astonishment, I had an acknowledgement of my submission *the next day*. I couldn't believe it. Years of getting used to the inhumane academic publishing model made me incredulous. Here was someone that took the time to acknowledge the time that I had taken to make this work happen, and it felt overwhelming, like an unexpected act of kindness that I was not quite ready to receive. The editor liked the project and offered to start the review process. She then announced a clear date by when the review would be done. A clear date! If it passed the review process, mere months after submitting my final draft, the book would be published in all e-book formats, would be free to download across a variety of platforms, and could also be bought—for a reasonable price—in paperback and hardback editions. It would carry a creative commons license, and I could choose among the different ones available.

This news—and the radically more humane way of treating people—couldn't sink in. Once again, I felt no joy. I couldn't believe it was happening, and not just because I wasn't used to it. It's because submitting my book to a new and radical press went against my training, and the anxiety of doing 'the wrong thing' swelled up and drowned the joy. After some time, I began to see that I had done the right thing. My book would be free to circulate, which is what I wanted, and I would be actively supporting a publication model that I strongly believe in. Will my book therefore not be recognized by my peers, by committees, by academic institutions? Have I jumped the line, doing something that only older academics with secure jobs are allowed to do? I have no idea, and I am working hard on not caring.

Since then, I have continued publishing chapters in edited collections that are invariably published with big, prestigious, ethically dubious presses. I am not above this and will probably never be. The process of unlearning is long, perhaps lasting a lifetime.

The 16-year-old that left Romania on a night train would probably look at me now and be astonished. So many experiences, so many places, people, ways of knowing, so much ignorance that I finally know I will never extinguish. He would be of course right. The migrant and academic life that I have so far led has been a privileged one, avoiding by sheer luck so many of the tragic detours that often sabotage the possibility of a good life.

I have become multiple, multiple times over, and by now I am committed to it. But this commitment, whether as a migrant, an academic, or a migrant academic, requires constant vigilance. There is a low-level force that pushes against multiplicity, be it in the form of personal belonging, academic allegiances, or ways of communicating with the wider world. It is like a slow waterway, seemingly tame, soft even, but with the tenacity to carve stone. Resisting being carved into one groove is the constant task of unlearning.

The forces working against multiplicity are not only tied to the migrant experience. They are part and parcel of academic institutional structures today. Perhaps migrant academics are a bit better placed to notice the process of flattening that these institutions tend to unconsciously engage in, because of their need to adapt, and the pressure to assimilate.

What I have written here is a personal thing, something that surely varies from person to person regardless of 'where they are from'. It would be absurd to claim that I speak for some universal category, like 'the migrant academic'! Far from it. Instead, I find it good to pause and identify some processes that are at play for everyone, but that become more easily seen when one is looking askance, by default. The process of learning how to be one thing needs to be called out, first and foremost for oneself, so that the unlearning can begin. Calling it out may also be one way of finally erasing the distinction between migrant and local; it offers a way to build solidarity, the most elusive thing in the academic environment today.

# (IN)VISIBLE INCLUSIONS AND EXCLUSION

# 4. Who Do the Dead Belong to? Considering the (In)visibility of Death as an Outsider in France

*Norah Kiereri*

I was at my parents' house in Thika, Kenya, in July 2021 for one of my usual Sunday visits. As I stopped and got out of the car to open the gate, I saw that a few meters down the road, there were vehicles parked on both sides. They were parked in a way that suggested that the occupants were being hosted at one of our neighbors' houses, whom I shall call Njambi. It was an unusual number of cars for a simple party on a Sunday; whatever it was, it was a significant function to draw this number of participants. My first thought had been a marriage ceremony, but those were hardly held on a Sunday. I asked my parents when I walked in if they knew what was going on at Njambi's place. They had not heard anything yet, but my mum noted that the vehicles had been there since Friday evening and had continued to grow in number. As we continued to muse over what could be happening, my mother received a phone call from the neighbor living directly across the road from us. 'What do you mean?!?' my mum shouted. Her whole demeanor changed. When she hung up, she reported that Njambi's mother had died on Friday. The vehicles we saw outside their gate were mourners who had come to grieve with them. As I left later that evening, my mum told me she would go for the 'prayers' at Njambi's house. The prayers involved singing and praying, a sermon by a pastor or representative of the church, and then fundraising and deliberations on the funeral arrangements. It didn't matter that COVID-19 was raging in the country

 https://doi.org/10.11647/OBP.0331.04

and in Thika; this is what church members, neighbors, friends, and family did for and with a family that had lost a loved one.

Let me take you back to 2020 for a minute. I had been living in the third district of Marseille since October 2019, when I joined the Aix Marseille University as an Anthropology/Sociology PhD candidate through the project SALMEA: Self-Accomplishment and Local Moralities in East Africa. When the COVID-19 pandemic broke out the following year, I was confined to my 15-meter-square studio on the eighth floor of a student residence. Despite seeing life on the street below me going on as normal, my phone was bombarded with news and figures that showed how dire humanity's situation was. Part of France's and the rest of the world's daily routine was reporting a collective daily count of new infections and deaths. The numbers were shocking, 25,000+ new infections in one day and 1200+ registered deaths in France alone! And in the following days, the numbers would be higher before they came down.

I was terrified at how many people were dying, but wait a minute! Where were they dying? Why did I not see evidence of this extraordinary number of deaths in my residence or city home to over eight hundred thousand people?[1] There was nothing unusual or out of place in the community around me, so who did the dead belong to? And were those people's grief and mourning visible? Not where I lived. I was not denying the reported COVID-19 deaths; rather, I was curious that I had not seen any sign of it. I was also not sure what I was looking for or what it looked like. I half-expected the sound of people crying in neighboring buildings to waft through my open windows like it would if I was in Kenya. I did not see a collection of vehicles or a gathering of people here in the third district. There was a lockdown in place, and that may have been the reason. Yet, even in the months before the lockdown, I realized that death was invisible to me in Marseille.

'Do the reported COVID-19 deaths in France also include deaths in Marseille?' I was unsure how to communicate my query to my PhD supervisor. I started by asking if people were dying in Marseille and saw the confusion on my supervisor's face. We were having one of our

---

1     'Comparateur de territoires commune de Marseille (13055),' Insee (L'Institut national de la statistique et des études économiques, September 22, 2022), https://www.insee.fr/fr/statistiques/1405599?geo=COM-13055.

regular calls via WhatsApp, which she made to check up on me; we could not meet physically due to the restrictions, and she knew that my socializing within my neighborhood and with work colleagues was limited because I could not speak French. I had become preoccupied with the apparent absence of evidence of death in the community around me. I was puzzled that it was invisible to me. In Kenya, I quickly realized, in contrast to what I was seeing in Marseille, death was experienced publicly by those who were bereaved and those around them. In the neighborhoods, there would be evidence of people congregating for the evening prayers—either the singing of hymns that drifted from the home to the street and neighboring homesteads or the swinging gate as people walked in and out of the home. It was also evident by the white tops of tents sticking above the fenced compound, betraying the shaded crowd that had gathered below. As with Njambi's mother's situation, the cars symbolized that something significant had happened. During my stay in Kenya in 2021, I remember being very aware of an increased death rate due to the significantly larger obituary section in the two main national newspapers. It was hard to ignore the funeral corteges that snaked through traffic, with the official videographer filming the entourage while sitting on one of the car doors with its window rolled down, and the hearse at the front leading mourners to the deceased's final resting place. Each car in the entourage would be marked with a red ribbon around the side mirror, as was the norm. Death was visible in a way that it was not in Marseille.

Back in 2020 in Marseille, my supervisor offered some possible reasons why death was not evident or visible in my community. Apart from the fact that my residence was nowhere near a cemetery or funeral home (at least to my knowledge), my supervisor also reminded me that most COVID-related deaths were happening in hospitals. Hospital or health officials might have taken over the responsibility of burying the dead in accordance with the pandemic regulations. Burial attendance was also greatly restricted due to the pandemic; when allowed, it was limited to family members. This made sense, but it did not explain why I had not seen a hearse traversing the streets of Marseille or its highways. It left me asking how corpses were transported from hospitals to mortuaries or funeral homes and then to the burial grounds. My supervisor explained that she was probably not the best person to provide answers to my questions since she had not experienced death in the family for a long time and she was not privy to any such occurrence among her work colleagues and friends. Her experience was limited. So, my questions remained unanswered. I wish to restate the reason for my questions here: the number of daily deaths reported in media were, in my mind such a significant number that I expected the immediate social impact or reaction to be equally significant. In my view, the life cycle of death as a social event was incomplete. I had not seen or had probably missed the indicators of the deceased's journey to their final resting place.

In September 2021, my mother passed away after being in the ICU for a month. Luckily, I was in Kenya since May of that year for fieldwork and deferred my return ticket at the end of August when she became ill and was hospitalized. I am grateful that I could spend time with her when she was healthy, visit and pray with her almost every day of her hospitalization, and finally be with family and friends as we mourned and buried her on her land just outside of Thika. A week before she died, I took my father for his check-up to the same hospital my mum was admitted. They had both been in the ICU, but he came out quickly and recovered his health completely. As I waited for him to finish up with his doctor, I sat down at the reception area with my laptop open, working on my fieldwork report that had a deadline, and determined whether I had received the payment for the fieldwork done in August. If I missed this deadline, I would have had to wait until the next month to receive my allowance, and would get it only if I submitted the report before the next month's payroll was prepared. My expectation was that the individual in charge of the process (and with whom I was in contact) would process my allowance pending my report, which I would submit once my personal crisis was over. Perhaps this was an overstretch of my expectations, but I believed that it was an arrangement I should have been able to negotiate. But it wasn't, and I needed the money, so I typed away in that reception room, waiting for my dad to come out so that I could take him to visit my mum in the ICU in the adjoining building.

A week later, my mother died. We buried her a week after her death. Before then, there were meetings every evening at my parents' house. My mother's pastors, fellow church members, former workmates, and fellow businesspeople attended the meetings every night along with relatives from far and wide. There was singing and prayers under a tent

4. Who Do the Dead Belong to?

whose top you could see over the fence. And there were numerous cars parked outside the gate along the road. I did not attend the meetings; instead, I remained behind at my sister's place, where I was staying for the duration of my mother's illness and after her burial. I did not cry in public except at the funeral, where I cried freely as I read my tribute to my mother. But my tears and pain were hidden behind my sunglasses and the mandatory face mask. I drove myself to and from the funeral. My car did not have a red ribbon, and I was not part of the cortege that escorted my mother from the funeral home to her burial place. Despite the visible ways I saw other people handle the death of a loved one, my personal experience was invisible to members of my family, friends, and neighbors. Not absent but hidden. I am aware that the way my experience with death was not absent but probably invisible to others is the same way that the evidence of COVID-19 deaths in France was not absent but hidden to me.

A few days after the funeral, one of my French colleagues, a senior researcher, suggested that I return to Marseille. She thought it would be better for me to come back and distract myself with a different environment and with work. I was baffled. My mother had just died. The human that made sense of the world for me and had continued to define my existence (even now, in my forties) was gone. The ground under my feet had literally opened, and I was free-falling through life in shock and terror—and this person suggested that Marseille and my work may do me some good. Rather than being in a familiar, socially safe place with family and friends, this person believed it was better for me to be in Marseille where she knew I had no friends and couldn't communicate with anybody because I didn't speak French well. Also, the idea that I needed distraction from this earth-moving crisis baffled me: was there any way to escape the pain that came with the death of a loved one? I still feel angry when I think about this. And I still struggle to make sense of this suggestion because what does it say about how the person perceived my mother's death and my loss? I find that this can lead me down a dark path because there are no good answers. Because I know her to be kind and generous, I reassure myself that she was trying to help. I do not think she was being deliberately insensitive or speaking out of malice. After all, people can be awkward when it comes to death. But at the back of my mind, I remembered the story a young Kenyan scientist shared at a friend's graduation party of his experiences working with Europeans and North Americans. He shared how the human resources policy on death stipulated that staff could take three days off if they lost a loved one and two weeks off if they had lost a pet. We laughed at the time; we were sure he exaggerated much of his story to make us laugh. His point was that Europeans and North Americans are extremely individualistic, and kin or social relationships are not as important as they are to Kenyans. I know this is not necessarily true; however, when I consider my colleague's suggestion, I wonder. Sometimes I wonder.

In most Kenyan institutions, one is entitled to about five days of compassionate leave to attend to the death of a family member. Additional days can be hived off one's annual leave. Also, one may negotiate additional compassionate leave days if one must travel outside town to arrange and attend the burial. I knew how to negotiate the days I needed from a Kenyan institution. However, I realized that I had no idea what my employer's policy was on compassionate leave at a French institution. Because I was already in Kenya for fieldwork for four months, I believe it was easier for me to stay on for an additional two months—that is, September and October. However, my contract does not allow me to be away from France for more than six months in a row, therefore I would have had to travel back to Marseille by the end of October. My supervisor, who has been my guardian angel in many ways, seemed to understand that I was not ready to come back and was contemplating deferring my studies. She advised me to apply for my annual leave, which would allow me to stay in Kenya until the end of the year. My leave request was quickly approved by the human resources official, who, in her email, also shared her condolences in one short sentence, 'I am sorry about your mum'.

When my mother died, I half-expected that I would see an email about my loss circulated to my colleagues by the lab administration. I did not tell the lab administration. 'But surely they must know about it?', I thought to myself. My experience with the Kenyan institutions I worked in was that the human resources sent out an email to the entire staff to communicate a co-worker's loss of a loved one. This allowed us not only to email out condolences and to contribute to the funeral expenses but also to appropriately welcome back the co-worker with a *pole sana* (Swahili expression for 'very sorry') and 'I'm praying for you and your family' when they resumed. I was not expecting contributions, but I expected that when I got back, I would receive the French version of *pole sana* and 'I am praying for you'. Was it that my colleagues did not know of my loss? Yet again, how were they supposed to know if I did not tell them? But how could they *not* know? I shared the news of my loss with two colleagues with whom I felt well acquainted enough to do so. It appeared that none of them shared it with the group. This has made me very curious about experiencing death in the workplace in France. I know that one of the two colleagues I had shared my news with is very reserved. She does not share her private life with the rest of the team; perhaps as an extension of her preferences for me, she kept my news private. Knowing my other colleague, it is possible that he shared the news with the department administrators. I can only speculate since I have not asked him about it. My own experience made me realize that during my time in the department, I had not seen a single email reporting the death of a colleague's loved one. But I had seen emails that reported the death of a former colleague. I still do not know what to make of this—the interaction between a bereaved person and his or her workmates in Marseille—because it is also invisible to me.

My experience with the demand for my fieldwork report to get paid my allowance while I was crisscrossing hospital corridors, and the expectation of my French colleague that I would travel to Marseille two weeks after the funeral made me believe that I had to put aside the loss of my mother and go on as if nothing had happened. It was one of my mentors, a resident in the Netherlands, that insisted that I stay in Kenya until I was psychologically well to leave. She reminded me that I had gone through a difficult month of crisscrossing two counties (Nairobi and Kiambu county) while dealing with the hospitalization of both my parents. She validated the fatigue I felt both physically and mentally, cautioning me that I could still be recovering from that and had not fully comprehended my mother's death. She alerted me that my stay in Kenya was not just for my sake but also for my sisters, who were younger than me and perhaps looked up to me as a figure of comfort. She demanded that I ask for a postponement of my thesis follow-up committee meeting, which was scheduled for the Tuesday after my mother's burial. She assured me that the university would allow my late registration because these things happen. She was adamant. I truly appreciate what she did for me. I think she understood how intimidated I was by the French bureaucracy,[2] which is often quite rigid and is daunting for an outsider who relies on Google Translate for most administrative and social communication. I believe she was also aware of the impact the perceived hierarchy between my French colleagues and me had on my assumptions and behavior. It helped that I had her as an ally, albeit in the shadows. She provided me an alternative voice and, specifically, a voice that could respond to the anxieties I had concerning what I saw as a rigid and hostile academic bureaucracy that I had trouble interacting with. I did as she advised. The thesis follow-up committee meeting was postponed by four weeks.

On reflection, I realize that the experience I detailed in the last four paragraphs was mostly my reaction to my imagination about what the French academic and work administration expected from me despite my bereavement. I was able to resolve the tensions concerning my university re-registration and my return to work and to Marseille. However, this would not have been possible without the intervention of mediators such as my French supervisor and my Dutch mentor, who were familiar with the workings of my institutions as well as my orientation, experiences, anxieties, and limitations. They not only mediated but also interpreted meanings for me—meanings that were often lost in communication via Google translations from French to English. They also explained or shed light on the cultural context and differences between my experiences and expectations and those of the people with whom I interacted. For example, I was not being offensive to my thesis follow-up committee members, whom I considered my seniors, by asking for our meeting to be postponed. Of course they would understand; were they not human too? Without the intervention of my mediators, I would have made decisions and done things I was not ready for, and probably my resentment towards my work and colleagues would have been unbridled, to the detriment of my studies. I am forever grateful to my supervisor, my mentor, and others who have been critical for my survival in Marseille as a Kenyan PhD student and a

---

2    The Oxford Learner's dictionary defines bureaucracy as 'the system of official rules and ways of doing things that a government or an organization has, especially when these seem to be too complicated'. I use the word here in this context.

French resident. I cannot forget the British professor on sabbatical here in Marseille, who, together with his wife, met with me online once every month in 2020 and 2021 to help me navigate my first academic year and the separation from my family during the pandemic.

I am still curious about how the French experience death. I saw my first funeral home in France in the town that I now reside in, Cassis, just outside of Marseille. In the days I have passed it on my way to the big mall, I have only once seen a group of about ten people gathered outside as if coming from or waiting to enter the establishment. I contrast this with funeral homes in Kenya that are busy almost all days of the week except for Sunday and maybe Monday, evidenced by the crowds that gather to observe the remains of their loved ones moved from the morgue to the hearse and the long line of cars parked both inside and outside the compound and beside the road, waiting to form the funeral cortege. Back in Cassis, the bus I was in quickly passed by the funeral home, so I couldn't make out if any of the people I saw had sad faces or were crying. I was curious about how they wore the experience of death on their faces. Perhaps they were looking for a kindred spirit in mourning like I was, unable to let go of their loved one, crushed by the terrible hand of death while trying to maintain a dignified posture.

It does feel like my contemplations about death in Marseille, triggered by the reported deaths at the height of the COVID-19 pandemic in 2020, have come full circle for me. I was aware of but could not observe other people's experiences with death in Marseille, and then I observed my friend and neighbor's loss of her mother in Kenya. The circle was completed with my own experience of death and my encounter with French responses to my loss.

The experience of death is perhaps not what many readers would expect to find as the subject of a contribution to a book on the academic experiences of foreign scholars in Europe. Yet, death has been a global preoccupation since the onset of the COVID-19 pandemic and has invaded our private spaces either through media or through our experiences and the experiences of those around us. In the paragraphs above, I have discussed my experience with death in the last three years, and shared some of my questions and reflections on the visibility and invisibility of death in my community in Kenya and in France. As Olga Burlyuk stated after reading a draft of my text, it is not that I am questioning whether the French mourn the dead; they do. My concern has been in the visible and invisible ways death is mourned. And in sharing my Kenyan neighbor's loss, I relay the expectations I had vis-à-vis what I observed or did not observe in Marseille. In sharing my own loss, I not only show how I did not conform to my own expectations of a visible performance of the activities linked to the death of a loved one, but also how I struggled with my anxieties concerning the perceived expectations of my French academic community as I dealt with my loss. I understand that because my worldview is shaped by my experiences growing up in Kenya, my perception of attitudes and practices in other countries may betray strong biases. These are not meant to be offensive; they are simply reactions to encountering the unfamiliar and reflecting on them, based on my worldview. I have attempted to relay my experiences and reflections respectfully to the communities in Kenya and France. Where I have failed, I ask your forgiveness.

# 5. The Invisible Migrant: The (Im)Possibility of Getting Behind the Iron Curtain of Western Academia as an Eastern European Academic

*Martina Vitáčková*

I did a double Master's, finished it in rapid time, and was awarded my PhD at the age of 28. Shortly after that, my PhD was published as a monograph. A bright career was awaiting me in academia, or so I thought. However, I did not consider that I did my PhD on the 'wrong' side of Europe. Even worse: I did not even do my PhD in Prague, which seems to be the only university in the Czech Republic that matters in the West. (Read: the only one they have heard of.) It made sense to me that I, even as a Prague native, would move to another side of the country. The Dutch studies programme was better in Olomouc than in Prague. And they offered me a full-time teaching position during my PhD, so it was the sensible thing to do. But I did not foresee the impact that this decision would have on my academic career. My PhD in theory of literature was part of the Bologna process, awarded according to the EU norms, with a former dean of the University College London as chair of the PhD defense committee, but alas! It was granted at a university located East of the former Iron Curtain. Around the same time, I fell in love and decided I wanted to live in Belgium. With the naïveté of a fresh doctor of philosophy, I thought the three letters behind my name

https://doi.org/10.11647/OBP.0331.05

mattered more than where I got the title. But in academia, just as in the housing market, location means a lot. Location and luck. Location and luck.

So I packed my books in cardboard boxes and relocated to Belgium, a tiny country crammed between the Netherlands and France, with three official languages and seven parliaments. The language would not be a problem, I thought, since I was proficient in one of the official languages and understood the other two. I did my MA in Dutch at Palacky University, Olomouc and wrote my PhD on Dutch and Afrikaans literature. I had also been teaching Dutch as a foreign language throughout my PhD studies to private and university students. I arrived in a country whose language, history, and culture I had studied at university level and had taught to many students. It was supposed to feel like coming home.

It did not.

I came to Belgium for the first time years before that. It was the summer of 2002, I was a first-year student, and I came by bus to attend a two-week summer school on Dutch language and culture, organized for international non-Dutch students who studied Dutch outside of the Low Countries (i.e. the Netherlands and Belgium). Part of the course was a home visit to a Flemish family for dinner. We went in pairs. I don't remember my fellow home visitor, neither where she came from, nor what her name was. The only thing I remember from the whole evening is the vicious xenophobia of the host family and their attitude of cultural superiority towards the two of us. Twenty years later, I still remember the shame I felt when the other girl and I were marched to the bathroom to wash our hands before dinner. 'That's how it's done here', the woman said. Afterward, she gave us a lecture on flowing hot water streaming from the faucet, which she thought we probably didn't have at home. We did. I recall being asked whether I knew what spaghetti was. I did. The lady never attempted to learn anything about 'us', so I didn't get the chance to inform her that we ate pasta at home as well. I would not have dared anyway, I guess. I was paralyzed by shock, and shame. I was also puzzled by the other girl's reaction to these humiliating utterances: she was smiling and nodding enthusiastically. Back then I was angry with her; didn't she understand that we were being insulted?! Now, I think she actually did not understand the language that well, and tried to be polite. Later I became angry with myself: I should have said something,

I should have defended our dignity against this horrible show of cultural superiority. Even now, after I have experienced thousands of such incidents—in private and work life—I still usually become muted by my own shame. I do not know what I'm actually ashamed of. Maybe I internalized the xenophobia I had been surrounded by for years.

Ten years later, I was willing to give Belgium another try, armed with perfect knowledge of Dutch and a university diploma. The welcome wasn't much better. When registering at the city hall, I greeted the lady at the counter, explained my situation, and provided my new address. The lady at the counter, whom I just had a five-minute conversation in Dutch with, looked at my papers, looked at my name with raised eyebrows, looked back at me, and asked in a slow, loud voice, 'Dooooo youuuuuu haaaaaaave a driiiiiiiving liiiiiiicense?' while making driving gestures with her hands as if she were turning an imaginary steering wheel. I did. And again, I didn't stand up for myself.

A few days later I was meeting a professor with whom I wanted to apply for a post-doctoral fellowship. While he really liked my research idea, he was worried about the quality of my PhD and wondered whether it was the same 'as the Belgian one'. It should be—Bologna, you know. But in practice, it isn't. My PhD diploma carries the name of an unknown university somewhere in Eastern Europe. Also, I had to have a full-time teaching position in order to survive financially during my PhD studies. Logically, I didn't publish as much as Belgian PhD students, who have employee status and a comfortable salary. So I tried to do another PhD in Belgium or the Netherlands. The problem was that, since I already had an EU PhD, no one would fund another one.

The cold shower of unacceptance is, oddly enough, connected with my knowledge of the local language and culture. It is also the thing that will get commented on the most in my everyday life. I am regularly complimented on how well I speak Dutch, usually in a voice of a parent whose kid just used a potty for the first time. After years of disbelieving and/or confused staring back, I am now able to reply that it would have been strange for me not to speak the language, given that I study Dutch and Afrikaans literature. Almost as often, people (and that includes colleagues in academia as well) point out that I still have a bit of an accent, don't I. In the eyes of these commentators, I do not fit the common image of an (academic) immigrant who still has to learn the language and customs of their new country. While it is completely acceptable for Flemish academics to be experts on British, German, or Japanese literature, the fact that I, an outsider, could have sufficient knowledge of the Dutch language AND literature seems to be beyond common understanding, even in academia. Perhaps if I studied Russian literature, since that is also in the East, or Czech literature, since that is written in my mother tongue... But the truth is that I know much more about Dutch and Afrikaans literature than about Czech literature. I try to follow Czech culture and literature from a distance. But my new Dutch/Flemish home culture and my specialization—Afrikaans literature—just take up too much time, and there is no space left for another culture. I am always happy when my Czech friends give me a book by a local author they personally liked, and that is just about all the cultural input I get. I am OK with that.

People are born, grow up, work, live, have families (sometimes), grow old, and ultimately die (always). Each of the stages can, however, happen in another country and/or culture. I, for example, was born in Czechoslovakia, grew up in the post-socialist Czechoslovakia, and after the 1992 split in Czech Republic (which since 2016 has used the official short geographic name Czechia), and had lived in Austria, the Netherlands, Belgium, and South Africa before I finally settled in Belgium. All these countries, spaces and cultures formed the 'me' that I am now. And frankly, I felt much more at home in South Africa than I ever felt in Czechoslovakia or the Czech Republic. After the years abroad, I now experience anything Czech with an uncomfortable mixture of longing, recognition, and unhomeliness. While I am Czech, and Prague-born, I cannot give you tips on good restaurants in Prague. I don't know what the most popular music is in the Czechia now, what the average salary is, or what the general opinion on global warming is. I do not know. I was born there, and my parents still live there. I know what my parents think and what those few friends I still have there think. But that is about it. I am as much a representative of the Czech Republic (pardon: Czechia) as Arnold Schwarzenegger is of Austria, or Jean-Claude Van Damme—the famous Muscles from Brussels—is of Belgium. I would fancy being called Brains from Bohemia, though...

And while we're at it, here are some more things I would really like to get off the table: I do not like Kundera. At all. I really wish people would stop asking me about Kundera. I don't know. See, I am a Dutch and Afrikaans literature scholar. And while *The Unbearable Lightness of Being* might be representative of Czechoslovakia back then (1984), it does not say anything at all about what the country and culture look like now. In fact, Milan Kundera writes in French these days, claiming he is a French writer now.

I do not speak Russian. I was supposed to learn that at school, but then the revolution of 1989 happened, the Soviet bloc collapsed, and the Berlin Wall fell. Learning Russian in a freshly freed post-socialist country was a big no-no, so I never did. Instead, I started learning English from a teacher whose English was hardly better than the students'. In fact, she was in the textbook exactly one chapter ahead of us. It is a miracle that this bumpy start did not discourage me and that I eventually mastered that language.

No, I do not know the Polish woman whom you are friends with. We immigrants do not all hang out together like members of some sort of a cult. Also, Polish and Czech are two separate languages, and speaking one of them does not necessarily mean you speak or even understand the other. Actually, I speak Dutch with most of my Polish friends because they are, just as I am, scholars of Dutch literature or language.

I am not a spokesperson for all Eastern European immigrants. And no, you cannot complain about your Polish plumber to me. And no, I won't feel any pride if you praise your Romanian cleaning lady in front of me. It sucks to hire a bad plumber, and good for you if you have found a good cleaning lady. The fact that we all come from the other side of Europe does not create a holy bond between us. That other side of Europe is not one country: it actually consists of many countries with their own languages and cultures that are not interchangeable. I would hope that university-educated people know that.

As a woman originally from Eastern Europe (because let's be honest: the term Central Europe is only used *in* Central Europe), many Western Europeans would expect me to be a cleaning lady. Or maybe a sex worker. That is just gendered xenophobia, and it needs to stop. When I moved in with my partner, many people, including some friends and acquaintances, made half-jokes that I was a mail-order bride. No one laughed. Many have insinuated that I was a gold-digger. At that point, we considered putting a house number plate out with Dr in front of my name and Mr in front of my partner's name. We have not done that. Yet.

Me speaking Dutch and being seemingly well adjusted to Belgian culture and society does not make me an ally to your xenophobia or racism. I would appreciate if I were not supposed to support the omnipresent Western European outrage about 'the immigrants'. It causes me outrage when I have to listen to that. And it hurts. Once I had to listen to a hairdresser complaining to me about all the immigrants at her child's school. There were too many of 'them' (read, 'us'!) to her taste, so she finally 'had to' put her child in another school. She wanted her child to learn Dutch properly. She expected me to understand and approve, as if I, of all people, would understand her concerns. But there it was again, the paralysis. So I just sat there, squirming uncomfortably in the chair, waiting for the moment when I could leave. I never came back. But I do come back to that situation in my head a lot, beating myself up that I should have said something, should have done something... Rush out with my hair half-cut, the hairdresser's smock flapping behind me like a superhero cape. I did not.

In Europe, whiteness is not homogenous, there are many shades of white, and not all of them are as privileged as it would seem from the outside. In fact, it took moving to South Africa to realize that I was white myself. I did not know. In Belgium, I am white, and my otherness stays hidden behind the fragile façade of my whiteness in many ways. I am the other, but not the visible kind. Neither my skin nor my hair are commented on, my clothing (even though sometimes frowned upon) does not disclose my origin... On the street, I am invisible, and my otherness stays hidden for as long as I don't make myself known. It only takes people finding out my surname or hearing a few words I exchange with my child for the façade to break into pieces. And there I stand, exposed in my otherness. My day-to-day experiences in the public space and in academia resonate so much with those of my fellow migrants who come from further away than Europe.

People hardly make an effort to pronounce my surname, some chuckle uncomfortably, some just call me by my first name. I am constantly asked about my 'home country' and culture. At the same time, people question the information I provide them in an act that can probably be coined as Westsplaining. I grew up there, lived through that time, the historical changes, but still, an average Westerner tends to think s/he knows better than I do. Because they went there on a city break. Or maybe read some

Kundera. Some days the emotional labor of keeping my wits together and not reacting to the never-ending microaggressions just consumes all my energy. My right to occupy the space, despite my Belgian citizenship (which I was finally granted after many years of living in Belgium), keeps being questioned. 'But you are not from here, are you?'

Even after having lengthy discussions with people, some just can't make the switch in their brains. They keep talking to me in LOUD, simple words, and short sentences, with lots of gestures. Checking whether I understand the most basic words. After all, I taught Dutch as a second language for years; I have multiple certificates to prove my proficiency in the language; I have written numerous articles in Dutch and on Dutch literature; and both my personal and work life take place almost exclusively in Dutch... But still, that question keeps coming back, haunting me, stirring up the good old feeling of shame for what I am. 'Do you know what spaghetti is?' 'Dooooo youuuuuuu haaaaave a driiiiiving liiiiiiicense?' I still do.

The imaginary Iron Curtain is still dividing Europe, and even the European Union is very much comparable to the wall of ice in *Game of Thrones*. It is so difficult to get behind, though not in the physical sense of the word. And once you are in, you are still considered a wildling without 'proper' schooling—someone that people should be mindful of. I would like to be able to say that the caution and cultural superiority that you are treated with stays outside academia, but that is sadly not the case.

I still have it easy: not being called out on my skin color, my hair, or what is covering it. My diplomas are, at least on paper, accepted. I can come visit my parents and my country of origin, if money allows, anytime I feel like it. I can fly to Prague, just waving my Czech or Belgian ID, walk into a bookshop and buy a Czech translation of Kundera. My parents can always come to Belgium and see their grandchild. But my 'easy' is also relative. While I am spared many microaggressions due to my 'white' looks, I also share the precarious state of migranthood, and migrant otherness. The feeling of never really belonging, of never being fully accepted. Even with my EU education, I am not always considered equal to my Western European colleagues. It makes me wonder if I ever will be.

# 6. Of Academia, Status, and Knowing Your Place

*Dragana Stojmenovska*

The day I started my PhD is also the day I stopped being a migrant and became an expat. September 15, 2016. That day, I went to the Immigration and Naturalization Service (IND) office in Amsterdam to pick up my residence permit, which was going to secure my stay in the Netherlands for the next four years. My expectations for how this visit was going to go were very clear. Walk in. Feel anxious. Exhibit socially desirable behavior. Sit down. Wait. Waiting room packed. Observe nervous leg tapping of others. Absorb anxiety of others. Look down at your hands and notice you are fidgeting. Worry you are not going to get the permit even though you got a letter that says you got the permit. Maybe you do something weird, and they say no. Maybe the civil servant accidentally drops the permit into the dark abyss. It is irrecoverable and they can't make you a new one. Your number on the screen. Your turn. Be nice. Show facial expressions that suggest that you, too, are fully human. Done. You got it. Feel happy about it and instantly reproach yourself for feeling happy (and thereby insufficiently anti-systemic). Go outside. The sun will be out. It's not. You are in the Netherlands.

I am in the Netherlands, and it has been six years since I moved to Amsterdam to pursue a liberal arts and sciences Bachelor's degree. Six years by actual count, three years according to the IND.[1] My regular trips to the IND during those years—to pick up residence permits—were

---

[1]	Years spent on residence permits of a temporary nature—such as student permits—count only as half-year periods towards the necessary time period for applying for a permanent residence permit or Dutch citizenship.

 https://doi.org/10.11647/OBP.0331.06

due to the fact that my home country, Macedonia (read 'Eastern Europe', 'Southeast Europe', 'the Balkans' or '??' for the purposes of this essay), is not part of the European Union. While this September 2016 visit to the IND was similar to previous ones in its sweaty-palms-inducing character, it was also different. A few firsts. For the first time, I was getting a so-called 'scientific researcher' permit, and for the first time 12 months were going to count as 12 months because this permit was of non-temporary nature.[2] And then, there was also one surprise: for the first time, I was in the wrong place. At the IND I was told that, to pick up my residence permit, I had to go to the *Expat Center* located in the *World Trade Center* in Amsterdam's business district. How very fancy! Walk in. Sit on a comfy couch in an empty waiting room only briefly. Get picked up by an enthusiastic smiling face. Would you like a drink and here is your permit and this is all you would like to know about it and how can *we* be there for *you*, Miss? Go outside. The sun is out. You turned from a migrant to an expat in just a bike ride.

In my research on gender and the workplace, I think a lot about the marriage of status beliefs about categorically distinct individuals (categorized on the basis of gender, race/ethnicity, migration status, educational attainment, and other axes of signification) and status associated with different types of jobs. Widely held social, cultural, and political beliefs about which groups of people are more status-worthy and competent than others interact with status beliefs about jobs to produce inequality in the initial distribution of jobs, as well as in the experiences within these jobs (Ridgeway, 2014). This shows clearly in my work on gender and workplace authority. Devalued groups such as women are under-represented in jobs that entail authority, positions which are generally associated with higher status than those that do not involve authority (Stojmenovska, Steinmetz, and Volker, 2021). The view on women as less status-worthy also influences their experiences when they do have authority at the workplace. Because of the perceived incongruence between women as a lower-status group and authority jobs as higher-status, women in authority experience hostile reactions

---

2    Non-temporary, but not permanent, because there are two types of non-temporary (niet-tijdelijke) permits, of indefinite (onbepaalde) and definite (bepaalde) duration, with scientific researcher permits belonging to the latter group.

from colleagues and clients in the form of harassment and bullying (Stojmenovska, 2023).

Much like most authority jobs, academic jobs in the Netherlands are seen as high-status jobs. Coming from years of precarity as a non-EU/ EEA migrant student and a working-class background (though academia got me into other types of precarity), my 'becoming an expat' story was just a preview of privilege. Over the following few years, I will have gotten to enjoy a financially comfortable life, traveling often to present my work and having the privilege of being seen as a legitimate source of knowledge at conferences and in the classroom. To call this merely 'a story of academia and status' is, however, not telling the full story. The more complete story—in my current narration of it—goes under the tentative name 'Of Academia, Status, and Knowing Your Place' and is about how (analogous to the way women are seen as incompatible with having authority in the workplace), my positionality at the intersections of migration background, gender, and class (among other things) is perceived as incongruent with being an academic in the Global North. Through recollection of a few social interactions I have had outside and within academia, I will speak about how these views, commonly held by the Dutch (and more generally, Western European) public, show up in interactions in everyday life.

## Interaction 1: "Coming from such a place"

It is a sunny Sunday morning, and I am at a friend's having breakfast. My friend is Dutch, and so is her flatmate. Her flatmate's dad is coming over to watch football with his son, a Sunday father-son tradition. Their favorite football club is playing; they are excited. As he walks into the living room, I make a mental note, something about football and masculinity and father-son traditions. My mind shushes itself: 'it's Sunday morning. Turn off any analyses of the patriarchy and refocus on the mundane, like that perfect medium-boiled egg on the table in front of you.' What is more mundane than the patriarchy, really?

I tell myself that I should not make any assumptions about the interaction I am about to have—I am meeting this person for the first time, after all—but my body starts feeling tense in anticipation. It is an embodied reaction I developed in response to microaggressions I have experienced while being in exclusively Dutch contexts, meeting the family and friends of my Dutch friends. I know it is going to happen. It happens *every single time*. Like this one time my friend's mother commented on how I probably can't afford a nine-euro bag—unlike her, who found the bag very cheap—at a time when I was working as a researcher at the City of Amsterdam, earning a decent salary. Or this other time when another friend's mother asked me, over Christmas dinner, in the presence of her Dutch friends, all with pitying faces, exactly how miserable my parents were.

I put away my well-founded assumptions and put my best socially appealing behavior on, asking about the flatmate's father's profession. He teaches at a high school in the Netherlands. I feel mild excitement about our overlap in professions, seeing an opportunity to connect. He does not ask about my profession, however. Instead, he *enquires* into my migration background, and gives the standard account on his experiences with 'that part of Europe'. How he once went to Bulgaria on a school trip where he met this teacher who showed him this traditional dance (note the return of the 'traditional dance' later in this essay). My friend interjects and says that I am a teacher too. Our interlocutor responds with little excitement, requesting the details. I explain that I teach social science courses to Bachelor's and Master's students at the University of Amsterdam, and that I am about to start supervising the theses of a group of Bachelor's sociology students. I notice myself trying to get through my sentences as fast as possible because something in the interaction makes me feel like I am giving unsolicited information. Then, it happens. His response: 'Oh, how special that *you* get to do this, coming from such a place.' I mumble something like 'yeah, special', and that is the end of this conversation.

While in real life I said one thing, in my head I wanted to say another.

Edit to my response to my friend's flatmate's father, the high school teacher: 'Yes, meneer, I do get to do this. As a matter of fact, I am extremely qualified to do this. Growing up, my mother worked in a textile factory and my father was a construction worker. Growing up working class and becoming middle class in my adulthood has taught me a lot about class, which is one of the subjects I teach. I also know a lot about gender, another subject I teach. Learned some new things after moving to your country, where I got to experience racialized sexism for the first time when the men I studied with said that Macedonian women have the perfect bodies and suggested I should bike to school naked.[3] This later got me into what we call 'intersectionality', another subject I teach. I have the lived experience but also got my books right. I had to work extra hard because I did not inherit the cultural know-hows on navigating (Dutch) academia from my parents. Add to this the fact that I needed a scholarship to study in the European Union, because your country's tuition fees for non-EU students are six times higher than those for EU students, and I was also not allowed to work to support myself financially because for that I needed a work permit. So, I got perfect grades in primary and high school, and continued working very hard in university to keep my scholarship and continue getting new ones. I graduated with distinction from both my Bachelor's and Master's and received a very competitive research grant to do my own PhD project. *That* is the place I come from.'

## Interaction 2: "Shouldn't you be elsewhere?"

There is time for informal chatter over drinks and appetizers after every seminar at work. I am chatting with two male colleagues who are more senior than me, one of whom is a self-proclaimed wine connoisseur and is giving an extensive commentary on the wine we are drinking and the different sorts of grapes. I am there and simultaneously in multiple other places, tracing back memories of the first fancy academic dinners I had and the way my eyes then carefully traced others' hand movements to learn which cutlery to reach for first. The other colleague 'jokingly' asks me if I shouldn't be elsewhere harvesting grapes, 'like the other Eastern Europeans.' I am taken by surprise and, in trying to compose myself, I am too slow to respond. Before I know it, the conversation is about something else.

> Edit to this interaction to include my response: 'Look at that, humor. Sociologists' preferred way of delivering -ist remarks (as far as I can tell). In using humor, sociologists intend to suggest that they actually mean the opposite of what they are saying, because they are sociologists and cannot possibly be classist/racist/sexist. Interesting, no?

---

3    Dominant representations of Eastern European women in the West—that have remained relatively stable over time—revolve around images of hypersexual(ized) gendered "others" (Deltcheva, 2005).

## Interaction 3: "Then maybe you should leave"

I am at a bar with a male Dutch colleague, having drinks. Two acquaintances of my colleague, both Dutch men, drop by. I am introduced as a colleague at the university. The acquaintances ask where I am from, after sharing their unsolicited guesses about where I come from. One of them imitates 'a traditional Macedonian dance' (there it is, the return of the dance!), after sharing that he had never been to the country and does not even know where exactly it is. They subsequently ask about my research. I tell them that I study women's under-representation in positions of workplace authority, after which they share their knowledge on the subject matter. They ask if one of the aspects I study is how women 'sleep their way up to authority'. They have heard this to be a rather common phenomenon in Eastern Europe. I make a quick exit to the restroom; I cannot be bothered to engage.

A few hours later, another male acquaintance of my colleague comes to the bar. The introduction goes in a similar way. After hearing what my research is about, this person expresses his surprise about me studying gender *in the Netherlands*. I wonder if the 'me' in the previous sentence should also be italicized. 'Coming from such a place.' Gender is, as far as he is concerned, not an issue in the Netherlands, he says.

> My response, unedited: 'Gender *is* very much "a thing" in the Netherlands, just like anywhere else. Depending on the indicator you look at, you will often find that the Netherlands is doing worse than other countries. My subject of research, known as "vertical occupational segregation" in the social stratification literature, is one example. For instance, if we look at the share of full professors who are women (the position of full professor being an example of a high-status job that involves authority), the Netherlands has one of the lowest shares of women full professors of all European countries.'

My interlocutor, unfit/unwilling/reluctant to engage in this conversation, responds with yet another classic: 'Well, if it is so bad here, then maybe you should leave after your PhD.'

# Pass it forward

Five years since my migrant-to-expat transition, the way being a migrant woman from a country classified as 'Eastern Europe,' 'Southeast Europe', 'the Balkans' or '??' routinely robs me of the higher status I would otherwise be enjoying as an academic 'expat' has changed little. What has changed, however, is that I am increasingly able to make sense of these interactions, to give them a name. Certainly, the sociological material in the few examples I engaged with is abundant.

These interactions are about who has the right to knowledge (re) production; who is to know, and who is to be known. My Dutch interlocutors—who are, by the way, white men who are older than me—express resistance toward me residing in the same body as someone who is teaching and doing research at a university in the Netherlands (Interactions 1 and 3). 'Coming from such a place,' I am someone who should not know things, and the suggestion that I *am* a legitimate source of knowledge is punished by telling me to leave (ehh, no thanks but you can pay for my ticket for the holidays if you like). I *cannot* know things but I *can* be known. And so my interlocutors can imitate 'a traditional Macedonian dance' without having the slightest idea of what Macedonian dances actually look like. I am tradition, and they are modernity. 'Gender is not a thing in the Netherlands'—and that pretty much sums up the dominant white Dutch self-representation as free of gender and racial hierarchies (Wekker, 2016).

Interaction 2 speaks volumes about class and race/ethnicity. By explicitly stating that I should be elsewhere, harvesting grapes like the other Eastern Europeans, my colleague is suggesting a few things. First, an ascribed and prescribed equivalence between being Eastern European and doing manual work.[4] Second, that because of this equivalence, I should not be working at the university, i.e., should be 'elsewhere.' Third, somewhat paradoxically, the humorous delivery of this message is supposed to soothe me so that I do not feel offended or embarrassed: I actually *am* an academic and so cannot possibly be

---

4    For context, note that jobs involving manual work in Western and Northern European countries are disproportionately occupied by Eastern European migrants, who are also among the lowest paid workers. See, for example, https://www.cbs. nl/en-gb/news/2019/14/nearly-180-thousand-jobs-filled-by-polish-workers.

doing work that is seen as inferior and less deserving of respect. Finally, my colleague uses humor as a means to detach himself of what is being said, assuming a shared understanding that being classist/racist/sexist is incompatible with being a sociologist.

In this sense, the 'knowing your place' part of the 'Of Academia, Status, and Knowing Your Place' story is also about having the toolkit to make sense of these interactions scientifically, which, I find, is immensely empowering. The stories that my interlocutors in these interactions tell themselves are not the only stories. They are also not the most important stories. Instead, I am looking at the stories tucked away in sociology books, those drawn from the lived experiences of migrants who came before us, the narratives that sometimes don't materialize into words in the space between me and the other person because I am too flustered, or trying to self-preserve, or have decided to pick my battles: the edits to my responses. I recall a conversation with one of my class/race/gender/sexuality course students a few years ago, during which she told me that learning about the dominant heterosexual dating script in the course has ruined her experience of dating men. I would not exactly claim that being a social scientist has ruined my experience of being in the world. Surely, as far as I am concerned, one is better off knowing about the script than not knowing about it. After all, it is not the knowledge of the script that ruins the experience, but the script itself. The downside of knowing one's place too well, however, is the state of constant anticipation that comes with it. As I write this piece, I am a week away from my Dutch students' graduation ceremony (where I will give graduation speeches and meet my students' families) and very aware of the pre-emptive analysis happening in my head. Will I get to hear 'one of those comments' again? How explicit will it be? What's the best way to respond? I suppose that this is my way of coping, trying to have control over the situation before it happens. The silver lining in all the analysis? Pin it down, pass it forward. Like I did here.

# Works cited

Cecilia L. Ridgeway, 'Why status matters for inequality', *American Sociological Review* 79/1 (2014): 1–16. https://doi.org/10.1177/0003122413515997

Roumiana Deltcheva, 'Eastern women in Western chronotopes: The representation of East European women in Western films after 1989', in *Vampirettes, Wretches, and Amazons: Western Representations of East European Women*, edited by Valentina Glajar and Domnica Radulescu (East European Monographs, 2005): 161–185.

Dragana Stojmenovska, 'Gender differences in job resources and strains in authority positions', *Gender & Society* 37/2 (2023). https://doi.org/10.1177/08912432231159334

Dragana Stojmenovska, Stephanie Steinmetz, and Beate Volker, 'The gender gap in workplace authority: Variation across types of authority positions', *Social Forces* 100/2 (2021): 599–621. https://doi.org/10.1093/sf/soab007

Gloria Wekker, *White Innocence: Paradoxes of Colonialism and Race* (Duke University Press, 2016). https://doi.org/10.1515/9780822374565

# 7. A Stroll through the Darkness: The Mental Health Struggles of a Migrant Academic

## *Anonymous*

This essay is written anonymously because putting my name on it would likely just be a never-ending source of anxiety. Why? Because mental health, in the eyes of many people, is still a reason for discrimination and a source of stigma. The reality is that mental health issues are so widespread that you certainly know someone who struggles with them. Our World in Data estimates the share of the global population with a mental health disorder to be at 10.7 percent.[1] British data from 2014 estimates that one in six people experience a common mental health problem within the space of a week.[2] US data from 2019 shows that nearly one in five US adults live with a mental illness. It seems these numbers are much higher than average in academia, as several recent studies have shown.[3] At an extreme, one of the surveys shows that '40 percent of PhD students based at UK universities could be at high risk of suicide.[4]

---

1 See, e.g., 'Mental health'. Published online at OurWorldInData.org: https://ourworldindata.org/mental-health

2 See, e.g., Sally McManus, Paul Bebbington, Rachel Jenkins, and Traolach Brugha (eds.), 'Mental health and wellbeing in England: Adult Psychiatric Morbidity Survey' (NHS Digital, 2014): http://content.digital.nhs.uk/catalogue/PUB21748/apms-2014-full-rpt.pdf

3 See, e.g., 'Exploring mental health in academia': https://www.technologynetworks.com/tn/articles/we-are-far-from-where-we-want-to-be-an-exploration-into-mental-health-in-academia-331273

4 See, e.g., '40 per cent of PhD students are 'at high risk of suicide', study says': https://thetab.com/uk/2021/10/14/40-per-cent-of-phd-students-are-at-high-risk-

https://doi.org/10.11647/OBP.0331.07

Unfortunately, due to societal stigma, lack of knowledge, misplaced shame, or other factors, many people do not open up about their struggles and self-doubts and do not seek help and treatment. So I want to open this paper by saying: if you struggle, you are not alone. You can find people who have been through the same situation and will support you, and professional help can do wonders. If you don't feel OK, and it is safe to get mental health care in your country, and it is accessible to you, but you are ashamed to ask for help because 'other people have it much worse,' or 'the psychotherapist will judge me,' or 'I am so broken, I probably can't be helped': please still try and ask for help. If you or someone you know is in serious distress or wants to harm themselves, call a crisis line or emergency services; there are useful lists of crisis lines in different countries online.[5]

My mental health struggles have been relatively mild compared to what many other people experience. I have struggled, sometimes a lot, but I have received abundant support from my social contacts and health professionals. I live in a country where I do not have to worry about putting food on the table, being evicted, or paying medical bills if I cannot work because of my mental health struggles. I do not have major caring responsibilities either. I am a linguistic and religious minority in my host country, but a majority in other senses: heterosexual, with stable residence rights. Fundamentally, I live in a country where mental health services exist and where it is possible to get medicine for mental health issues, which is not necessarily true in other parts of the world. Therefore, if you feel that my struggles have been relatively mild compared to yours, it probably is so. On the other hand, if your struggles do not seem quite as bad, it does not mean they should be discarded either.

There are several factors which, in my opinion, pose mental health risks or an additional mental burden for migrant academics in the Global North. My arguments draw closely on my particular experience of studying and conducting research in a few Global North countries and the insights I have obtained from reading about and engaging with others in similar circumstances, but they are likely incomplete. The

---

of-suicide-study-says-226001

5    See, e.g., Wikipedia's list of suicide crisis lines: https://en.wikipedia.org/wiki/List_of_suicide_crisis_lines. You can also call a general emergency number operating in your country, such as 112 in the European Union or 911 in the US.

'local' academics face mental health issues like the migrants and the newcomers, particularly if they too have to deal with discrimination and continuous assessment. However, the experience of relocation and integration into a new society may serve as an aggravating circumstance or maybe even a cause. So, without further ado...

I feel that one of the main challenges of being a migrant academic with mental health issues is that critical thinking is literally part of your job. As an academic, you are mostly alone with your thoughts; you try to concentrate, reflect, and create new ideas. You are probably very successful in identifying weaknesses in arguments, doubting the established dogmas, reflecting on the limitations of your approach and methods, and creating new theories. Unfortunately, this very skill can make you highly self-destructive. It has happened to me countless times: as soon as I sit down, open the laptop and try to do some work, my brain decides it is the right time to recall some previous trauma or mistake, try to resolve some anxiety-induced doubts, or worse. These self-critical thoughts, which can escalate into self-hate, can be of a more personal nature or they can be work-related, as you worry about your productivity, evaluations, and the uncertain future. It is easy to enter a downward spiral where you cannot work because of your mental struggles, and then your struggles are further aggravated by the fact you are not 'being productive.' Admitting to your bosses or colleagues that you are struggling with sensitive personal problems or have been unproductive for the last two months can seem (or actually be) daunting, as they may be cold, dismissive, or think you are 'unfit for academia.' On the other hand, struggling with your demons alone is incredibly isolating and scary, and this is where being a migrant plays a huge role.

When you move countries, inevitably, a lot needs to be done, and often you have to do it alone; even if (a) family member(s) is/are tagging along, you have more responsibility towards everyone. Whether you are a single person or part of a family, most of us need to feel connected with broader society. I have felt very acutely how isolation is bad for my mental health. Now think about a migrant academic trying to integrate: it is not easy in any circumstances, but even worse if you are an introvert, or if you do not speak the language of the majority in your new country, or the local people are reserved, or you work long hours as it often happens in academia. Your previous experience may also have an isolating effect. Maybe you want to talk about the issues in your home country which no one except you understands or cares about, or you are used to dressing simply or maybe just cannot afford the very polished and refined way in which locals are dressing, or everyone around you goes skiing every year, and you have never stood on skis before. It is easy to feel 'out of context' in a new environment. Your attempts to do extracurricular activities to get better integrated may bring you together with a group of other expats, which is nice but does not necessarily help you get integrated or acquire valuable local contacts. Relocating with a family may help you feel less isolated but may also prevent you from meeting locals, as well as bring other unique challenges. And the next thing is profession-related isolation because science is often done in solitude, and moreover, some environments can become quite toxic, with researchers aggressively competing amongst themselves. In my case, I spent many evenings and many office days *completely alone*, sometimes talking on the phone or texting with friends abroad. Many people only experienced this for the first time during the lockdowns for the COVID-19 pandemic and struggled massively, but for many other migrants and me, that was reality for a while. In fact, COVID-19 might make us all more empathetic to the struggles posed by loneliness and social isolation, but not many people empathized before that (or even now, after it). There has not been enough recognition for the additional precarity of migrants who live in further pandemic-induced isolation.

To be honest, it has been not only difficult but also plain irritating for me to struggle with the added impact of mental health issues, all the while trying to fit into the new place, deliver, and just be like everyone else. I see it as an extra burden: you cannot quite empathize with your colleagues and other contacts who complain about their 'ordinary' problems or 'just' the logistical difficulties of moving when you must *also* fight the mental health fight. In general, it is not very easy to explain a mental health issue to someone who has never experienced anything similar. Therefore, in addition to struggling, you also have to choose the right words to help the other person understand what you are going through. This does not really help with isolation.

In addition to isolation, which means lack of positive human contact, there is also discrimination, which, in turn, means negative human contact. In my experience, these can go together or separately. I have personally not experienced much discrimination, but I am also quite good at trying to blend in. I have experienced structural discrimination against foreigners—for instance, in relation to rent and language issues—and some discrimination of a more personal character. In my case, this did not contribute much to my mental health issues, but still, it dampened my level of optimism somewhat. Other migrant academics obviously have had it much worse, not only in the foreign environment in general but specifically in their workplaces.[6]

When you migrate, you often need to reinvent yourself. Many mental health issues, at least in my case, have been caused or aggravated by low self-esteem. Back at home, I had learned to cope 'decently.' It is highly likely that if you made it to the Global North as an academic from the Global South, you have already achieved something in your country of birth, built a support network, and felt like a 'somebody.' All this can be easily nullified when you move 'upwards.' You may need or want to reinvent yourself to fit the new circumstances, or at least I felt that I had to do that. Reinventing oneself may be a positive experience if you get back in touch with what you want and see that your wants can be satisfied in a new setting. It can also be rather negative, especially if you need to prove your credentials all over again, because your previous achievements may not count, especially if you have not studied or worked in the Global North before. In such cases, you have to rediscover or create new skills and abilities that will make you competitive in the foreign environment. In any case, rediscovering oneself is not likely to go smoothly, just like the process of scientific inquiry is normally not linear. You will stumble and meet dead ends on the way. The additional problem for a person prone to mental issues, at least in my case, is that this process of self-discovery and rediscovery may trigger old traumas, and dead ends will aggravate self-esteem problems. I had to go through a painful and time-consuming process of self-reinvention, which was partly triggered by external events but partly necessitated by the requirements of the new place.

The previous points sound challenging, do they not, but now add another specific feature of an academic job: harsh and continuous assessment. For most academics who do not have permanent positions

---

6    See, e.g., 'On being excluded: Testimonies by people of color in scholarly publishing', https://scholarlykitchen.sspnet.org/2018/04/04/excluded-testimonies-people-color-scholarly-publishing/.

(i.e., tenure), migrants or not, this is coupled with precarity: you only keep your contract (and thus, your means to live) if you keep delivering, delivering, and delivering results. Delivering results in academia is not so straightforward either. You fight against several external factors, particularly funding and journal review times, where a paper can easily take two years to be published. Moreover, you fight against the academic culture of assessment, where it is virtually impossible to submit a piece of work, however innovative and strong it is, and not get many suggestions for improvement. Constructive criticism is good, but it often gets rather destructive in academia. The reviewers often feel like they have to demonstrate their intelligence by nit-picking, or assert themselves by asking an author to rewrite the paper in line with *their* point of view. Talk about demoralizing and inducing self-doubt! So much has been said already about the scarcity of tenure, fierce competition for academic jobs and grants, and academic publishing that I will skip repeating it here. Some added difficulties for migrant academics are that they may come from environments where certain skills (for instance, academic writing) are taught differently. Some risk having to emigrate again, elsewhere or back to their birth countries, if their performance is found lacking and their contract is not renewed. Ultimately, instead of taking some time to adjust and deal with the realities of your new life, as you would be able to do in an ideal world, you have to hit the ground running and often keep working beyond your normal working hours to deliver the much-needed results. I see the relationship between the culture of continuous assessment and mental health issues as a potentially vicious circle. Mental health issues can prevent you from publishing or getting grants, for instance, if you cannot concentrate for prolonged periods, but lack of achievements also aggravates the mental health issues.

Among all of the ups and downs one has to face as a migrant academic, it is easy to forget about self-care or slip into denial of your mental health difficulties. There is always the next chapter to write, the next presentation to prepare, the next project application to write, the next paper to review... Taking care of your mental health relies on support networks that you may not have immediately available as a migrant. Healthcare also requires time, money, and enforcing borders in your personal and professional life, and you may not be in a position to afford any of those. As a migrant, you often face extra hurdles in getting financial, linguistic, or administrative help. Denial can be an 'easy way out.' Unfortunately, I think that denial is not a *sustainable* way out, but I believe that it will get better if you work on it.

Many people in the Global South would probably like to study and conduct research in the Global North. Unfortunately, my path as a migrant academic in the Global North has been much darker than I would wish for anyone. Thankfully, after several years, I think I have finally managed to reach a sort of a relatively stable stage. To quote JK Rowling, 'rock bottom became the solid foundation on which I rebuilt my life,' at least to some extent.[7] This has been possible thanks to receiving mental health care, support networks, being able to make some other life improvements, and a lot of reassessing and re-evaluating myself. Moreover, I have decided that, in the future, I will try to pursue a career outside of academia, specifically to reduce the mental load I have been facing due to precarity and other specifics of this field. This decision in itself has brought me some inner peace. Yet I am still far from being happy and secure in myself. And unfortunately, so many people right now are facing similar issues to mine, or much worse. As Rowling also said, 'I had no idea then how far the tunnel extended, and for a long time any light at the end of it was a hope rather than a reality.'[8] I sincerely hope that we can evolve towards greater understanding and greater solidarity, but for that, people's attitudes and the structure of academia itself needs to change.

---

7    JK Rowling, *Very Good Lives: The Fringe Benefits of Failure and the Importance of Imagination* (Sphere, 2015).

8    Ibid.

# BORDERS, MOBILITY, AND ACADEMIC 'NOMADISM'

# 8. Eighty Dates around the World: On Gender, Academic Mobility, and Reproductive Pressure

*Maryna Shevtsova*

I am 39. In the last nine years, I have lived in three continents, eight countries (in case you are curious, these are Ukraine, Hungary, Germany, Turkey, Thailand, the US, Sweden, and Slovenia), ten cities, and some 20 to 25 flats. I speak five languages fluently and can express myself quite well in four more. My best friends are scattered around the globe: in typical suburbia in Florida (US), EU headquarters in Brussels (Belgium), a residential area in Dnipro (Ukraine), and somewhere next to Zurich (Switzerland). They all have kids, and their mobility is, therefore, limited. This means that I should schedule my vacations and long weekends more carefully if I want to keep those friendships alive. I also need to visit my parents in Ukraine regularly, and, luckily, that's where one of my best friends lives, too, so it's a combo! You could probably hire me as an expert on how to move smoothly and start your life from scratch in a new country. I would charge you a lot, though, as my future flat mortgage will not pay itself—unless you are one of my fellow migrant academics, but then you probably know all those things better than I do.

When I am not struggling with typical academic anxieties—a long list of unfinished papers, nasty comments from 'Reviewer 2' on the article I submitted to that journal four months ago, and nights spent over an endless funding application—I actually find my life interesting, entertaining, and, I dare say, intellectually challenging. I travel a lot

   https://doi.org/10.11647/OBP.0331.08

and could afford some mobility even during the pandemic, as Sweden (where I ended up in 2020) did not have any lockdowns. My circle of friends is very diverse, and I am lucky to have very supportive and loving parents. I have never been poor. I always had a place to live and good food in the fridge. I have almost never been unemployed. I might not be able to recall when I had my last real vacation, but that's part of another story. Most importantly, I happen to have a job I really like! I am a scholar and researcher working on the topic of LGBTQ rights and gender equality in Central and Eastern Europe. I am also working as a diversity consultant for NGOs, international organizations, and the private sector—a job which pays well (even if it is demanding) and is, actually, a fun and rewarding task as you feel like you are changing the world for better (even if that change is tiny so far). By now, you are probably wondering what my essay is doing in an edited volume on migrant academics' precarity, like this one. Am I not supposed to be complaining and telling you all about the hardships of my academic post-PhD life? Bear with me; we are coming to that.

## How it all started

I grew up in a family of university professors; my mom defended her PhD in economics when I was a toddler, and my grandmother did her habilitation (second dissertation defense) when I was seven. They both were department chairs (my mom, in fact, has stepped down just this year, being in her early sixties) and have worked in academia all their lives. If you have watched 'The Chair' on Netflix—well, this is what their lives looked like, only the salary was ten times lower. In our family, the words 'our child has to have good education' never meant 'have a BA from a good university,' it actually meant 'have at least one PhD.' This came together with yet another conviction: 'working in academia is the best kind of a job for a woman as it is well-paid, respected, and allows you to have a good work-life balance.' If the latter makes you laugh, don't: it was true, indeed, in Soviet Ukraine in the 1970s-1980s. Provided you did not mess with the Communist Party, teaching at a university meant you had a nice flat, two months of paid seaside vacation, and a rather comfortable working schedule.

Then the 1990s came, and with them the collapse of the Soviet Union—and the collapse of the old system of education. By the time I was about to graduate from high school (1999), Ukrainian universities had lost half of their staff simply because salaries were so low that one could barely survive teaching at three universities at a time. Those who stayed either could not find themselves a place in the new market economy or were enthusiasts who really believed that academia was their destiny. Some of them, like my mother, were also lucky to have a spouse or partner who provided for the family financially, so they could just work there for the sake of work. Interestingly enough, then—and to some extent even now—for a man to have a wife or daughter working in academia in Ukraine was considered prestigious: it meant that you could afford it.

When the time came to choose a university, my family was gently pushing me towards the department of economics where both my mother and grandmother worked. I was never good at math, though, and I loved foreign languages and travel. A compromise that we found—international economic relations—had something to do with economics (mostly just the name, as I quickly realized) and offered two foreign language courses instead of one. I managed to add Spanish to English and French soon and could not have been happier!

By 2004, done with my MA, I found myself in my very first personal crisis. I did not want to work in academia in Ukraine. It did not pay well, it was half-destroyed, and it lacked role models for me. I was gathering the courage to leave the university for good, feeling totally prepared to work in export-import operations and earn enough to feel independent and cool at the age of 22. I considered applying for a scholarship abroad, as I had always dreamt about spending a year or two in a better-quality academic setting, and I applied for MA in international relations at the Central European University (CEU), Hungary, and Edmund Muskie Program in the US. I got short-listed for interviews but did not make it to the final cut. Now I know that, had I prepared a bit more and reapplied the year after, I would have had a very good chance of being selected. I did not do so, however, because—here it comes!—I was almost 23 years old, the year after I would be 24, time to get married and start a family, so no point in wasting time traveling for yet another MA degree. Instead—good daughter that I was—I started a PhD program in my Alma Mater to please my mom; and to earn a living, I got myself a full-time job with a large export-import company.

I will spare you the details of the next five to six years of dissertation writing and failing to fight corporate world sexism, and will introduce you to Maryna facing her second personal crisis. Being 29, I could be considered somewhat of a career success story in my city: a deputy purchase director of a big company and an assistant professor at a major university. By 2012, we had some economic growth in the country, and academia was actually recovering. I was still not-so-happily single and without kids: not that I wanted to get married or have kids at that point, but according to the larger part of the Ukrainian society, my career success could be easily explained away by the mere fact that I had failed as a woman! I wasn't fully satisfied with my success story either: teaching international economics was hardly my passion, and having a responsible job in a large company was less pleasant for knowing that my male colleagues were paid two and sometimes three times more for the same work—and sometimes even for working less.

Being almost 30, I thought I had nothing to lose. I first considered doing a post-doc abroad—but soon, to the huge disappointment of my mom and myself, I discovered that my university degree was not competitive at all in the Western universities that offered funding. I was also not sure that a longer endeavor like a PhD was a good idea; I knew very little of how Western academia functioned back then anyway. Somehow, I came across information about the gender studies program at the CEU. I still don't know what I was thinking, but I applied for a one-year MA program, having figured out that if I got the scholarship and used what little savings I had, I could afford it—and I was accepted! And so, a month and a half before my 30th birthday, I departed to Budapest with two big ambitions: to change my life completely and to learn Hungarian. The first came true; the second failed miserably.

## Living a dream?

Leaving Ukraine being almost 30 and unmarried (mind you: being divorced by 30 is still actually considered *better*), I felt extremely awkward when I had to explain to people that I was going to study again. I tried to change the topic so as not to tell them what exactly I was going to study because I vaguely understood then that gender studies had something to do with... women's rights? Feminism? Non-discrimination? I was unable to explain how this could be translated into any kind of future employment, so I preferred not to go into details. I simply invented the version that this was some kind of gaining additional qualifications abroad. I later found out that my parents actually thought that I was studying psychology and that I would be back to both my jobs in a year.

At the CEU in Budapest, however, I discovered that there was a world where my 30s could be easily turned into my new 20s! It was acceptable to be 30 and single, it was expected that you had no kids, and moreover, it was OK to do an MA in gender studies. However, gender studies were stigmatized by many students even in such a liberal university back then. I remember being told things like, 'you are too hot/ too normal/ too nice to be from the gender studies department.' I hope CEU students are better than that by now.

Anyway, nine months at the CEU taught me a lot about myself. In fact, I'd learned so much that I dared to apply for a PhD at exactly eight universities across Europe. Seven turned me down. Then, three months after the graduation ceremony, when I'd already landed a journalist position on a business TV channel in Kyiv (don't ask!), an official letter from Humboldt University came. I got a full scholarship for three years of doctoral studies in one of the best German universities! I was going to Berlin!

These days, whenever I talk to younger students applying for a PhD, I try to do something I wish somebody did for me: if allowed, I offer them an honest account of what my life during and post-PhD looked like. Because back then I had no idea. I chose to call this section 'Living a Dream?' because this was how it felt to me most of the time. However, I am pretty confident that many people could call the same experience 'Living a Nightmare,' and they would be right, too. My three years of PhD had their ups and downs. When you are 33–35, your peers start buying flats and cars, but you can only afford shared accommodation. You eat in MENSA (student cafeteria in Berlin) and drink cheap beers, stay in hostels when traveling, and can't afford many things that people who chose 'normal' jobs after the university can. Sometimes when my Ukrainian girlfriends were discussing in our 'self-support WhatsApp chat' how they negotiated six-digit salaries in Big 4 companies, I felt awkward and tempted to start sending my CVs to Ernst&Young and Deloitte. But then I remembered my days in the corporate office—full of calls and meetings I hardly cared about—and I did not.

You are also frequently quite alone on your PhD journey; my supervisor gave me extremely little support, and I barely had one 30-minute consultation per year with her (oh, German academia!). My graduate school had a counter-productive attitude: we were constantly told stories about how we should not count on finding jobs, how precarious academic life was, and how it was publish or perish, so many students stopped trying to be friendly and started seeing each other as competitors. There was no career support or mentorship program and, being a student from a foreign country and a non-German speaker, I had to struggle on my own to figure out the complex rules and norms according to which German higher education and research institutions function. Looking back, I remember having nightmares about being unable to finish the dissertation and consequently failing to find a job. I also had a feeling that I did not belong. I needed to take additional courses during all four years of my PhD to catch up with other students who had BAs and MAs in political science in Germany. My German was not good enough to maintain conversations with colleagues during lunches. Whoever tells you that you do not need German to live comfortably in Berlin as this is 'such an international city'—don't believe this person!

Yet, I still lived a dream. I am, for one, convinced that to be doing a fully-funded PhD is a privilege. You are given three to four years of paid time to read, learn, travel, and do research on a topic that—should you have chosen wisely—you deeply care about (mine was on LGBTQ activism in Ukraine and Turkey). I made wonderful friends. I met people I respect and admire. I traveled. I learned. I grew. When I am asked advice on whether to do a PhD, I try to stress that while doing a PhD offers you things, it also takes much away from you. It requires a lot of self-discipline, thick skin (I still take criticism with so much pain), and hours of psychotherapy for many of us. Was it worth it? Some days I am positive it was. Some days I am not entirely sure as I have too many questions in my head.

# Eighty Tinder dates around the world

Academic careers in the modern world are infamous for their precarity and instability; after all, this volume is dealing exactly with this topic. Nevertheless, let me explain to you why I still chose to pursue an academic career.

I have a Ukrainian passport and hardly a marketable profession anywhere except Ukraine: even if a degree in international economic relations sounds 'international', you soon realize that there are too many local professionals in other countries for a company to want to pay for a work permit for you. In other words, my options to move abroad were minimal. Suppose I wanted to relocate to a specific country. In that case, I could probably look for an international company with offices in my country and try this way. But what if I wanted (and it happens to be so) to try *living* in multiple countries during my lifetime? Then the pool of professions that offer you such a possibility—in which employers are fine with obtaining work permits for you, you do not need to learn the language of the host country, and you are still paid decently—gets rather small. IT industry is one option, but I am not good at coding, unfortunately. Academia is another, and while the whole spirit of academia is about making you feel like you are never good enough, I am convinced that at least I am a better scholar and researcher than I am a programmer. Academia actually encourages mobility: the more jobs at universities worldwide, the better, as both your geographical expertise and ability to work in a multicultural environment (and teach international students) grow. In my field of social sciences it also offers you a flexible schedule, though (of course) sometimes it means you are free to choose whether you prefer to work 24/7 at your university office or from any other place on the planet Earth, but that's, again, another story. And it pays you to write on things you actually care about (like this piece, for example). It all comes at a price, obviously. I argue here: the price is always higher for a woman.

Remember I told you at the beginning that I am an expert in moving smoothly? I know how to pack for a month, for half a year, for a year; what Facebook groups and Telegram channels to join to stay updated; where to find life hacks on such basic things like opening bank accounts, finding accommodation, and paying utility bills. Other (no less essential) knowledge that is in my possession is how to date internationally. I moved ten times in the last nine years, and that's approximately how many six-to-twelve-month-long relationships I have ended—and started again. In between, I was going out on dates for coffees and hookups, and I must say that dating applications are the easiest way to establish a new social circle once you move to a new country or city. I found out a long time ago that not all people on these apps look for lifelong relationships or one-night stands. You can find good friends there or simply people to show you around, tell you more about the new city you will call 'home' for a year or two, and introduce you to their friends or colleagues; in other words, people who will make your life easier and nicer overall.

The first month (or even two) after the move are always a huge stress. Even with much moving experience, you need to figure out thousands of things that differ from country to country, and you can never foresee what kind of an emergency will happen. In Germany, I was promised to be paid my salary for the first two months upon arrival—'to help me settle down.' However, I needed to open a bank account first, for which I needed a valid address, for which I needed to have a flat. It is already challenging to find a flat in Berlin, especially if you do not have a credit story *and* a bank account, for which you need a flat—you get the idea, right? Not to mention that you have to pay your first month's rent and a deposit when you still haven't received your salary. Then, when you magically collect all those documents and bring them to the university, it takes them almost a month to process them. All in all, I received my money at the end of month two—two months later than I was promised! Had I not had my savings and my parents' support, I would not have been able to survive these two months in Berlin. I know several people who had to ask their parents to buy them tickets home because of this.

Then, once the anxieties of the first months are over, you start socializing actively and going for dates and meet-ups to build a new social circle for yourself. As I wrote above, dating apps do help a lot. I also do not believe that friendships are made only when you are young: it is all a matter of time and effort invested. While I agree that the Danes are much less likely to befriend foreigners than the Spaniards, you can usually succeed in establishing a cozy circle of friends, especially in bigger cities. In some countries, other migrants like you will prevail; in others, more locals will be open to befriending you. Needless to say, the most painful part comes with the end of your contract and moving to another country. Some friendships are just not meant to be maintained on distance and, unfortunately, neither were 'most of my romantic relationships. More or less with the end of each work contract or fellowship came the end of another love (or just sex) story of mine, and I should admit that in most cases, I was the one who heard, 'I am not ready for a long-distance relationship' from the other party.

## Questioning my ways

In my early 30s, with my international dating experience, I was a welcome addition to conversations with both my Ukrainian friends, happily married or divorced, with or without kids, and international friends, mostly young professionals, half of them also on the dating market. As you might know, dating applications are places where you can meet all sorts of people, and some dates can be a particular experience. Some of them are even painful, but you can always make a party anecdote out of it afterward. You deal with cross-cultural, cross-religious, and cross-professional differences, sometimes extremely different dating cultures and expectations, starting from whether to split the bill or not and finishing with when it is considered appropriate to first have sex, as well as with cute or scandalous misunderstandings as either one or both of you are not using your first language. What I intend to say here is that being a young working woman professional *and* single and dating was considered OK when I was under 25 in Ukraine—closer to 30, I was clearly frowned upon—and refreshingly OK again in the countries to the west of Ukraine when I was under 35. But as I grew older, I discovered that liberal attitudes in Western countries also have their limits, especially if you happen to be a woman.

I have chosen to leave Ukraine, among other reasons, because there, I felt like I had no time to try to be something else except being a mother and a wife. I felt like I had failed at both missions. I had this time abroad, but only for several more years. At 35 and older, I felt like all the choices I had been making had to be questioned next to one *big* question: having a stable monogamous relationship and, sooner rather than later, a kid. 'What is wrong with you?', I was asked, being 29 and single in Ukraine.

Now the same question—'what is wrong with you?'—comes when I am 39 and single in Western Europe.

What is wrong with you if your longest relationship lasted no more than a year and a half? What is wrong with you that you know so much about Tinder and one-night stands in different countries? What is wrong with you actually *being* on Tinder? What is wrong with you that you actually *want* to move again and again? Are you running from something? I cannot tell you how many times people told me this 'deeply philosophical' phrase that 'you cannot escape yourself'.

It seems that there is one comfortable picture of a successful life in the minds of many of us: a settled couple of young professionals with a kid or two, nothing like digital nomads, those 'weirdos' teaching yoga or surfing on Goa, or Instagram influencers. A 'normal' person is not supposed to want to be changing countries and, of course, every woman is expected to be looking for 'the one,' a romantic story to have. And if you are single again in your pre-40s, everyone will hurry to ensure you that it is because 'the one' is about to come and maybe 'this is why you have to change so many countries, because somewhere *the one* is waiting for you.' Yes, exactly, you got me; this is why I am doing this!

I have been working with the topic of LGBTQ rights in quite a conservative society since 2013. When I started posting work-related texts and videos on my Facebook page, unexpectedly, people I had not seen for a decade or so started writing me private messages asking me questions like 'how come you have the money and the possibility to travel so much?' and 'oh, and by the way, did you change your sexual orientation?' I hesitated each time between telling them to mind their own business or explaining to them that one does not 'change' their sexual orientation as this is not a choice. Sometimes I got angry and sometimes amused how desperately random people needed an explanation on why I lived the way I did.

Do you know what still provokes a much stronger reaction from people than talking about gay rights? Child-free women by choice! It is very difficult for me to understand why in such an overpopulated world, people are still so obsessed with the idea that women choose not to have children, but you would be amazed to read some of the comments of my compatriots under the videos or articles on the issue.

I am not sure if I am child-free by choice or by chance; I might try to have kids later or adopt. And I also have to question now whether my being single is by choice, because some would interpret this as 'no man wanted to continue being with me.' My gender clearly has to do with this. In so many couples women follow their male partners abroad as the men are pursuing their careers; the opposite happens so much more rarely. My male colleagues neither have that biological clock ticking, nor people around them constantly reminding them about their limited childbirth opportunities. Finally, a man traveling for work is generally seen as a successful nomad, while a woman traveling for work is often seen as the one without stable foundations in her life, escaping something, or—even worse—desperately looking for a husband from a richer country. Yet I am pretty sure that I am a traveler by choice—and by *my* choice only.

I wrote this piece because I am convinced that women who follow not-so-traditional ways—even if their ways cross nobody's borders—still seem to bother our society, which, deeply bothered by our choices, makes us question ourselves all the time. What is wrong with us? Why are we not fitting in? Maybe we are not trying 'hard enough'?

So when in doubt—yet again—over all those past choices, I remind myself of one thing I know for sure: I am in academia and I have lived in different countries, having made a very conscious decision. And I plan to live in several countries more because this is something that makes me really happy—not because I can escape, but rather because this way I learn more and more about the only person with whom I have and will have a lifelong relationship: myself.

# 9. Have You Ever Heard of British Hospitality? Neither Have I

## *Vjosa Musliu*

It is April 2017. I am working as a post-doctoral fellow at the Free University of Brussels in Belgium, within the department of political science. I have recently been invited for a research stay of two months at Warwick University in the UK. It is my dream department, and I could not be more excited. My husband, a researcher at the Catholic University of Leuven, will accompany me. My university is paying for all the expenses of the trip, including the stay and the accommodation.

Though we are residents in Belgium and employed at Belgian universities, I only have a Kosovar passport and my husband has a Turkish passport. This means we have to undergo the excruciatingly long visa application—like most citizens of the Global South have to do.

'I hate this!', I say to my husband as we rush to take the train in Ghent to go to the British Visa Centre in Brussels. Even though this may well be the 100th time I have applied for a visa, every single time I have the same reaction: edgy, angry, and about to blow up. As I walk, I occasionally pad my belly to remind myself of the bigger picture and that it's just another horrendous visa procedure. I am five months pregnant and expecting a baby girl.

As we leave the train in Brussels South Station and aim to head out, we see that the exit we are headed to is blocked by Belgian soldiers, who have been patrolling regularly ever since the terrorist attacks in Brussels in 2016.

'This is insane!', I say yet again as we make a detour to go through another exit. I am holding a giant binder containing all the documents required by the Visa Centre: my Kosovo passport, the letter from the UK

   https://doi.org/10.11647/OBP.0331.09

university hosting me, the letter from my current university in Belgium saying that I actually work there and I am not a fraud, ten pages of my bank statements to prove that I actually get paid on monthly basis, a letter from the dean of our university proving, once again, that I work for the university and I am going to the UK for research purposes only, the documentation of our accommodation in the UK, the return ticket from Brussels London, and proof of payment for the visa application worth 380 pounds. My husband is holding a similar binder with a certificate of our marriage, a letter of motivation that he will accompany me while I do my research stay, a letter from his university that says he is employed as a post-doctoral fellow at a Belgian university, ten pages of his bank statements, yet another copy of our accommodation in the UK, and the proof of payment for his visa application worth 380 pounds.

Breathing heavily, we finally arrive at the gate of the Visa Centre. I hit the buzzer.

'Do you have an appointment?', asks the person via the intercom.

'Good morning. Yes, we have an appointment at 10:20. My name is Vjosa Musliu.'

A couple of seconds later, the door opens up and we take the elevator to the second floor of a five-floor glassy building. On the second floor, there is only the British Visa Centre, outsourced to a private company called TLSContact. There is another giant glassy door to get through. My husband hits another buzzer and we wait there. A man in his late 30s comes near the glassy door and asks us, yet again, whether we have an appointment. I repeat my name again and indicate the timing of our slot.

The door opens up and we are directed to a waiting room filled with people. I take a look around and see many 'Eastern Europeans' with their passports in Cyrillic; many more people are from the Middle East, and there are a handful of people from sub-Saharan Africa. Waiting rooms of Visa Centres in Western (European) countries always look the same to me. They are like clubs composed exclusively of 'barbarians.' I find a chair to sit on, take a sip of my water and pat my belly. My husband sits next to me.

On the wall in front of me, there is a corkboard. On top of it, there is a banner, printed in color, that says: 'Welcome! British Hospitality'. Below that, there are easily 20 pages in black and white unpacking British hospitality. On the first page, there is a list indicating the prices for a tourist visa, student visa, and family reunion visa. The next page is filled with warnings: 'You cannot prolong your stay while in the UK'; 'You cannot reapply for another visa once in the UK'... The next page explains at length the limited category of people who are entitled to seek asylum in the UK. As I read that, I have an urge to both scream and burst into hysterical laughter all at the same time. I hold myself and instead grit my teeth and clench my fists; a smirk slips away.

The same man in his late 30s who opened the door for us comes inside and hands us yet another document we have to fill in. Again, the same personal details asking about our names, passport numbers, and reasons for visiting the UK, just in case we have forgotten since we filled out the excruciatingly long application online. After we fill in the document, we are called into the 'application room.' Unlike the waiting room, this is a smaller and darker room. There are three cubicles with three workers processing applications. I go first to the cubicle in the middle and hand in the pile of my documents. The worker goes through them meticulously as she double-checks everything with her computer.

'Can you put your hand on this device please?', she asks after she seems to have filed everything. 'We need your fingerprints.'

I put the four fingers of my right hand down first. Check. I put the fingers of my left-hand down second. Check. Then both of my thumbs together until the green button is lit. Check again.

'Your application is complete now. You will receive your passport with a decision on your visa at your home address within two weeks,' she says politely.

My husband goes through the same procedure as I wait for him in the waiting room.

***

Less than two weeks into the application, my husband—who is to accompany me on my research stay—receives his passport with his three-month visa. No sign of my passport.

Twenty days since the application and I still have not received anything from the British Visa Centre. Before this one, I may have easily applied 30 times for visas to mostly Western (European) countries. I have experienced every 'visa issue' in the book: from being refused a visa because I 'am too young' (USA), to my passport being deemed illegal because Kosovo is not a member of the United Nations (China), to not being able to travel alone and unaccompanied by a man (Iran), to my file being lost and not processed on time (Austria), to receiving the wrong visa and being called on the spot to reapply (Belgium), to receiving the visa only a couple of hours before my flight to the final destination (Switzerland), among others. Given my track record, I am naturally worried.

In the meantime, the hosting university in the UK is making final arrangements for one of my first guest lectures. I still have to prepare for that guest lecture but I have been too busy stressing about the visa. We have to be in the UK in less than three weeks.

It is a Tuesday and I am having my regular seminar class on conflicts at the Free University of Brussels, where I work. Today, we are discussing one of my favorite authors, Doreen Massey, and her seminal work on spaces and places of othering. Ironically, a student from Iraq links Massey's work with the border politics of the European Union. While she does this in a compelling academic fashion, I can see how much of her knowledge on the topic is embodied, as she might have gone through similar visa procedures to me in order to come and study in Belgium. Unlike usual, I am sitting at my desk and discussing with my students spread out in the large classroom. It is early afternoon and my belly feels particularly heavy during these hours. Halfway through the lecture, I see a British number calling me. I would normally never take a call and interrupt my class, but I know this is something major. I excuse myself from the students and head out to take the call.

'Madam, there is a problem with your passport. Would it be possible for you to come on Friday again for a new application?', asks a woman from the British Visa Centre.

'What do you mean there is a problem? I have to file a new application from the beginning, again?', I ask in disbelief.

'We made a mistake when we registered your fingerprints so we have to do it again. You have to pay 380 pounds again but we will reimburse you because this is our mistake,' she continues calmly, and asks again whether Friday morning would work for me.

Angry and reluctant, I agree to yet another visa application for Friday morning. It is not as though I can do anything else.

After my class, I call my husband to tell him about the situation.

'So, the British Visa Centre called me....', I say and wait for him to take his guess on what could have possibly happened.

'They won't give you a visa because you will pollute the pristine British air?', he asks as he chews his dinner.

'Close, but no,' I reply, waiting for yet another guess.

'They won't give you a visa because they liberated your country and now you are just being a greedy Balkan woman?', he asks again, sipping on something.

'They made a mistake in my application. So, I have to file a new one. Again!', I reply, almost screaming.

'Oh, I am sorry, beba. That's worse than my two guesses combined,' he replies, and reassures me that we will file the application together and that he will gather all the documents for me.

***

It is Thursday evening. One non-alcoholic beer for me and a Trappist beer (ale) for my husband, we are sitting at our dining table filling out a new visa application. I open a new account.
Username.

I insert.

Password.

I insert.

'Password is too weak,' says the page.

I insert another one.

'Password must contain at least one capital letter,' says the page.

I insert another one with a capital letter.

'Password must contain at least one symbol.'

I insert a new password with an exclamation point.

'Password must contain at least one number.'

'Oh, fuck me!', I scream and I reach for the beer glass of my husband. I take a sip of the cold Trappist and insert a long password with an exclamation point, many capital letters and a number, hitting the keyboard loudly.

'Did you take all your anger out on that password?', asks my husband.

'I sure did,' I reply, and hand him the laptop to do the rest.

'Let the fun begin,' says my husband as he starts to fill in the questions[1] for me.

*'What is your gender, as shown in your passport or travel document? Male, female, unspecified?'* He reads the question out loud and then fills in the answer.

*'What is your status? Single, married, separated, widowed?'* He reads the next question out loud and fills it in.

I sip more of my non-alcoholic beer.

*'What racial identification do you identify as?'*, he reads and then he theatrically turns towards me. *'White? Non-White? Black? Hispanic? Indigenous? African American? American Indian? Alaskan Native? Asian Indian? Asian/Pacific Islander? White Non-Hispanic?'*

'How is this even legal?', I ask in disbelief as if I am seeing these questions for the first time.

'I was not finished,' he says as he scrolls down.

*'Native Hawaiian? White Caucasian? Non-White Caucasian? East Asian?'*, halfway through he stops reading. He clicks 'White' and moves to the next question.

*'What is the ownership of the place you currently live in? I own it, I rent it, other'.* He reads the question out loud and fills it in.

*'What permission do you have to be in Belgium? Temporary visa, permanent resident, other?'* He reads and fills in the question, yet again.

*'How much do you earn each month after tax?'*, he asks and reaches out for my bank statements to fill in the sum.

---

1    The questions below are not fictional. They are retrieved exactly as they are given in a British Visa Application form.

*'Do you have another income or savings? How much money do you have in savings?'*, he reads again and checks on my bank statements to fill in the sum.

After 20 more questions about taxation, travel, birth certificate of my parents, marriage certificate of my parents, we move to the next set of questions.

*'In either peace or war time have you ever been involved in, or suspected of involvement in, war crimes, crimes against humanity, or genocide?'*, my husband reads the question out loud and ticks 'No'.

*'Have you ever been involved in, supported or encouraged terrorist activities in any country?'* He reads the question and ticks 'No'.

'Wait! During the 1990s, like all Albanians in Kosovo I was charged with terrorism by the Serbian government. Thou shalt not lie in a visa application,' I reply.

'Sure,' he says dismissively and moves on to the next question.

*'Have you ever been a member of, or given support to, an organisation which has been concerned in terrorism?'*, he reads and ticks 'No'.

I shake my head in disbelief and grit my teeth.

*'Have you, by any means or medium, expressed views that justify or glorify terrorist violence or that may encourage others to commit terrorist or other serious criminal acts?'*, he reads.

'No, but after this application we might,' my husband replies himself this time and clicks 'No' yet again.

*'Have you, by any means or medium, expressed any extremist views?'*, he reads out loud and we both burst into laughter.

'Cheers!' We make a toast and then he clicks 'No' yet again, and the laughter ensues.

*'Have you ever engaged in any other activities which might indicate that you may not be considered to be a person of good character?'*, he reads, widening his eyes and wearing a cunning smile.

'I stole a bike when I was 12,' I respond as I reach out for some cashew nuts.

*'Is there any other information about your character or behaviour which you would like to make us aware of?'* He reads the question theatrically.

'Yes. I think it's insane that you conquered half the world and your national dish is deep-fried fish with chips!', I reply sipping more of my non-alcoholic beer.

'Beba, that's racist,' my husband says, laughing out loud.

'Oh, yeah! I am the one to be sued for racism here,' I reply.

We print the long application letter. My husband assembles all the other documents from the bank, the city hall, and my employer. The next day I go to the British Visa Centre in Brussels. I give my fingerprints again, hand in my passport, and pay an additional 380 pounds. One week later, I receive the passport with my visa in it. In less than one week we pack everything and leave for the UK for two months.

\*\*\*

While in the UK, I had a wonderful time at Warwick University, and we absolutely loved Scotland.

I am now back in Belgium, eight months pregnant, and I look like I am about to pop open anytime. I spend most of my days trying to reach the British Visa Centre—outsourced to a private company called TLSContact. It turns out, they never reimbursed me the 380 pounds, which they were supposed to do immediately, given that they made a mistake while filing my application.

On their website, there is neither an email address nor a phone number that you can use to reach them. Researching for hours, I find a hotline that seems to be connected to their office. I wait in line for hours. There is no answer. I do this for days in a row. There is no answer.

During the exam period at the university, one day I decide to drop by the Visa Centre in Brussels and show up unannounced. I wait at the front door until the next 'barbarian' comes for their visa appointment. When the buzzer opens the door to let them in, I smuggle myself inside with them.

'I am here to inquire about the reimbursement of my visa,' I say to the man in his late 30s who opens the door of the Visa Centre on the second floor.

'You cannot come here without an appointment,' he tells me as he stands in front of me, not letting me get inside.

'I cannot make an appointment because there is no option to do so if you are not applying for a visa,' I respond.

'Why did you not call?', he asks, stoically standing at the door.

'There is no phone number or email. I have been calling for days on that hotline. No answer. This was your mistake. You should have made that payment long ago,' I reply.

'Take this number and call Nicolas in Paris,' he says as he gives me a business card with a phone number handwritten on it. 'Our headquarters are in Paris. He can give you an appointment.' He abruptly closes the door.

I am livid. Livid and thirsty. I go downstairs and buy water from the vending machine.

I sit at the corner of the hall and give a call to this Nicolas in Paris. No answer.

Unable to reach Nicolas for days, I return to the British Visa Centre yet again the following week. Yet again, I smuggle myself inside after the receptionist buzzes another fellow 'barbarian' in.

At the glassy door on the second floor, I see again the same man in his late 30s. He is not happy to see me, which in turn makes me happy. With a smile on my face, carrying my gigantic belly, I approach the glassy door.

'Nicolas has not been responding to my calls. And the money has still not been paid by your office,' I say.

'I don't have staff who can deal with your file right now,' he says and prepares to leave.

'Either let me in or I will wait here until I give birth in this very corridor,' I say with my smile intact.

Across the glassy door, he mumbles something to himself, which I imagine are words of care for me and the child I am carrying, and lets me in.

'Please go to the waiting room. Laura will see you in a minute,' he says and disappears into the hallway.

Half an hour later, Laura comes to the waiting room to pick me up. She has a British accent, speaks French fluently, and looks East Asian to me, but her skin complexion is white. 'I wonder in which racial category she would fit were she to apply for a British visa,' I think to myself as I follow her to the small and dark application room.

Among the three cubicles in that small room, the one next to the door is the only one free. We sit across from each other. Her computer stands in between us. There is barely half a meter distance between the cubicles so you can hear all the conversations of the applicants with the personnel. The couple in the first cubicle is from Afghanistan. The woman with a child in the middle cubicle is from Russia.

'I need to enter your application online in order to deactivate it,' says Laura to me. 'Can you please give me your username and your password?'

Upon hearing that, the little room suddenly became a little bee hive from where I had the urge to run.

'Can I retrieve my application on my laptop?' I ask her, unwilling to give her my username and password.

'That is not possible due to security issues,' she says. 'Just give me your username and your password and I will deactivate it for you. Then we can make the reimbursement,' she adds carelessly.

'Can I come to your desk and fill in my details?' I insist further, unwilling to divulge my login details.

Laura looks at me with suspicion and moves away from her desk to let me pass. Narrow as it was, I could not pass along the cubicle with my huge belly.

'Look, it will be way easier if you just give me your details. Your account will be deactivated right away anyway,' she says and sits back in her chair. I go back to my initial seat.

'Username?' she asks, and looks me in the eye.

'Vjosa Musliu,' I say, and prepare myself for the next.

'Password?' she asks again.

I hesitate at first. I look at her, clear my throat and say: 'UK...fuck you, you ugly pieces of shit... exclamation point, 2017,' and swallow right after.

It is pretty obvious that the other two workers, the Russian woman with her child, and the Afghan couple all heard my password.

Laura is slowly typing the password. In the process, she lifts her gaze but does not look at me directly.

'It says the password is wrong,' she says, looking at me this time.

'Ah, sorry. 'UK' is in capital letters...and so is FUCK YOU...both times,' I continue, as I swallow with difficulty out of discomfort.

'OK, I'm in,' she says.

Two minutes later and after a lifetime of stares from the other two workers in my direction, Laura deactivates my account.

'It is deactivated now. You should receive your money in a matter of days now. We are sorry for the inconvenience,' she says as I collect my bag and my water to head out.

In the corridor, I see the Afghan couple again. They both giggle and give me a thumbs-up.

'Good luck with the visa,' I say to them, smiling.

'You too,' they say, smiling back.

***

Three weeks have passed. I am nine months pregnant. The British Visa Centre has still not paid my money. Unable to reach them through any means of communication, I alert the university administration, explaining to them in detail what happened. The Ombudsman's Office is appalled to find out that there is no way—no phone number, no email—to reach this Centre in the event of a complaint.

Next, I reach out to the Belgian federal police and the legal office for national consumer protection to inquire for advice. It turns out the British Visa Centre is not liable to Belgian authorities. The only way they would be able to intervene is if the Visa Centre refused to give my passport back.

In desperation, the head of my department sends an official letter of complaint, in the name of the department and of the university to the British Ambassador to Belgium. I file another letter of complaint in my own name and send it officially to the British Embassy in Brussels, too.

A week later, we get a response from the British Embassy in Brussels—a polite nothingness— indicating that the British Embassy is not responsible for visa services and that, in fact, these services are conducted by TLSContact, a private company contracted by the British Foreign Affairs Ministry. If it ever existed, it seems that British hospitality has been outsourced to a private company with headquarters in Paris, where neither the Embassy itself nor the 'benefactors' of that hospitality can seek accountability in cases of damage.

***

It is March 2023. The UK is out of the European Union. My daughter is five years old. I still have not received my money back from the British Visa Centre.

# 10. On Being a 'Migrant Academic': Precarious Passports and Invisible Struggles

## Tara Asgarilaleh

Speaking of institutionalized and systemic inequality, I have definitely spent more time on visa applications and appointments and completely pointless and humiliating procedures than on university and grants applications together.

Not a long time ago, I read these words by a friend,[1] and it made me think of my own experiences and of so many other colleagues and friends whose stories of movements, crossing borders, visa applications, and permit requirements reflect inequalities that are unfamiliar to some, but which have become part of the lived experiences of those who carry what I call 'precarious passports'. In the beginning, I used to think (naïvely) there was something wrong with me, as I faced troubles in almost all my visa applications—in particular, in those aimed at Europe and North America. It did not take too long before I noticed that I share these struggles with many fellow students and researchers in a similar position to mine.

Being an academic can be a highly precarious position in itself, in a context of hyper-competition, insecure contracts, and all the uncertainties that come with them. The precarity, however, varies enormously depending on where one is based, including which country

---

1   I would like to thank my friend who kindly allowed me to refer to their words in this piece. I do not mention their name as they preferred to remain anonymous.

   https://doi.org/10.11647/OBP.0331.10

or which institute. Being a 'migrant academic' and holding a precarious passport adds another layer of precarity to the livelihoods of academics who carry these passports, such as myself. By 'precarious passports', I mean passports that have been rendered invaluable, inferior, or even a security threat due to broader geopolitical forces embedded in neoliberal and neocolonial globalization processes. Passports are mere objects. However, they gain or lose value and meaning in accordance with societal and geopolitical relations. This is not to deny certain privileges that come with being part of academia, which allows for access to spaces and things that I could not have been part of without having such membership. For instance, being a member of a prestigious university gives me access to various institutional resources, activities, and events. These are just some examples of privileges, material and non-material, that come with institutional memberships. Being a part of the academic environment has enabled me to navigate certain institutional structures that I could perhaps not otherwise afford—for example, endless bureaucratic paperwork procedures, various applications (such as long- and short-term jobs), and visa and grant applications. However, by acknowledging my privileges I do not undermine the struggles that I and other 'migrant academics' encounter as a result of having precarious passports—in my case, an Iranian one.

I shared my visa struggles once with a professor at a university, hoping to receive some support in what I was going through. In reply, they said: 'But you are not alone; many other people are experiencing this, and you should not let this distract you from your project.' I felt paralyzed that day. My visa could have been withdrawn at any time, which would have affected my entire study program. I was told to just focus on my project because I was not the only one going through the experience. I wondered whether this would have been any different, for instance, if I had a different nationality. Whether I would have received a different kind of support. Through time, I have found out how my experience could have been different, when I heard about other students' experiences with their professors—those who carry privileged passports—for whom my story of visa complications was an unfamiliar one. Privileges tend to become invisible easily, especially when we do not make an effort to be aware of them.

Albeit unemphatic, my professor was correct in one thing: many people carry precarious passports. And not all of them can focus on their academic work or studies, distracted as they are by continuous visa hassles and systematic border inequalities. That is why my story matters. While it is a difficult story to tell, I have decided to share it, because it reflects such great yet invisible inequalities that exist in our institutions, that keep reproducing themselves, and disrupt a more just path in which academic knowledge can be produced, accessed, and exchanged, sometimes simply by creating walls of silence or negligence, or through the lack of any form of empathy.

I first moved from my home country, Iran, to the Netherlands in 2015. Due to a major administrative delay, I was informed later than expected about my funding. I faced a one-month delay to my arrival to the Netherlands. My visa process at the Dutch Embassy under the student visa procedure went quicker than I imagined. Having been granted a full scholarship by my university, along with family support—including (but not limited to) financial support for my visa application, and my own savings from a part-time teaching job during my bachelor's—definitely played an important role in facilitating the expensive process. However, the entire visa process application was still at least as lengthy and time- and energy-consuming as my admission and application process, and possibly more complicated. I faced a similar, even longer delay of three months—and a much more complicated process—while moving to the UK in 2019 for my PhD, despite having been granted full funding for the entire project, the absence of which could have made an even more serious barrier to the visa process. I noticed this considerable difference in how things could have gone with my moves to the Netherlands and the UK when I began to chat about this with some other international students at my institution, the majority of whom were from Europe and North America and experienced much smoother processes.

Visa hassles often do not stop when you are granted initial approval for your visa status. They continue affecting you in various ways. Firstly, it is about when you want to arrive at a place for the first time and receive a first-time entry visa. For instance, for a person carrying a precarious passport, the amount of work and visa requirements is enormous compared to when you carry a privileged passport. Yet despite this extra work, the possibility of rejection or a considerable delay for a visa is much higher. If granted first-time entry, it is about navigating regulations on how best to ensure that your visa stays valid. In this way, the anxieties involved in taking care of your visa become an important part of your decision-making processes in conducting research, constantly counting how much time you must spend in each place so that your visa(s) stay valid. Secondly, there are mobility-related issues when you want to cross further borders as part of your academic path, because having been granted entry or temporary residence in one region does not grant you access to other locations.

Due to the delay in my Dutch visa and my late arrival to the Netherlands, I missed all the introductory events and activities that could have helped me familiarize myself with the new environment. Thanks to some of my great fellow students and teachers, I did not feel as lost or lonely as I had expected during my arrival in Amsterdam, considering that this was such a big change for me, from the very mundane everyday life to the educational system I was not familiar with, including the English language (in which I had never studied previously). The delay in my arrival to the Netherlands was only the beginning of all my visa struggles. In fact, crossing borders as part of my academic life has been anything but a smooth process. I have always paid what Bathsheba Okwenje (2019) calls 'emotional tax', on top of other costs, material and otherwise, which often result in great exhaustion and frustration, distracting me from the work I wish I could enjoy.

When I graduated from my Master's in Amsterdam, my access to conferences was disrupted several times due to my nationality. I could not present and participate in a major conference held in the US at the time, despite my abstract being accepted, due to the so-called 'Muslim Travel Ban.' Although a letter criticizing this ban was written by the conference organizers, the fact that the conference was held in the US in the first place—where the ban prevented nationals of seven countries from going—was upsetting to scholars and researchers like myself. We also experienced a lack of actual support or empathy from the conference organizers, and no appropriate alternative means of attending was provided, despite it being among the major conferences in the field. I was even charged the full registration fee, regardless of my absence being out of my hands. In the beginning, following my own inquiry, I was told that I could present my work through alternative online means. However, this did not materialize. At the time of my presentation, the panel organizer wrote me at the very last minute that they could not host me due to technical problems, and hence, I was not able to join the panel after all. Although technical issues happen during online events, the conference organizers' lack of appropriate communication and accountability following what happened was highly disappointing. When I wrote to request a refund, I was told that it was my problem that I could not join the panel. Refunds were only possible in cases of medical emergencies. The lack of recognition of why I could not join in the first place, due to the so-called 'Muslim Travel Ban,' and later, due to the technical issues—neither of which was in my hands—was highly disturbing.

I decided to make a complaint about the lack of refund to the conference organizers. I received a refund in the end. However, this was not a smooth procedure. During the entire process, I often felt lonely, as it was primarily me reaching out for support without receiving any expressions of solidarity from my colleagues. I decided to make a complaint anyway—to commit myself, my time, and energy—despite it keeping me away from the work I wanted to do instead, hoping that doing this would reduce the chance of it happening again in the future (Ahmed, 2021). I must note that, during the complaint process, a good friend—who is a senior researcher based in a different institute but in a similar field to mine—brainstormed with me. He had gone through a similar path regarding the consequences of the so-called 'Muslim Travel Ban.' He knew other researchers with similar visa struggles wanting to attend the conferences held in the US at the time. It was heart-warming to think it through together and to navigate such a disconcerting process not entirely alone. Having this support from a friend was especially precious because we lacked any form of solidarity from any department in our institutes, and from our colleagues, who traveled to the US and participated in various conferences in our unwanted absence. In a sense, as much as we can imagine complaints as non-reproductive labor, as Sarah Ahmed puts it, 'it can also be a hope, an aspiration, it can be what you have to do to breathe. Sometimes you complain to survive. However, this does not mean that you get through' (ibid.). For me, it was both. However, sometimes one simply cannot afford to complain, as what has happened to you is already burdening and exhausting. One might not always have enough resources and capacities to afford to do so, or might actively not want to make a complaint in order to avoid encountering any further painful experiences.

After graduating from my Master's program, while I was applying for post-graduate positions, I was rejected for a vacancy in a big project.

I was alerted to the call for this position by a colleague/friend who knew I was looking for a position and told me that the vacancy fitted my profile perfectly and that I should apply. I wrote to the primary investigator requesting feedback. In reply, she wrote that she was really sorry and mentioned my nationality as a main concern in not inviting me for an interview, despite me being a potentially good candidate. I wrote back and expressed my enthusiasm for the project. I wrote that I reckoned it would be a pity that I would not be able to be considered a candidate due to my nationality, especially if I was considered a strong candidate. I never got a reply to this last email. I was devasted. This was similar to other reactions to my nationality and hence, was not really a surprise. But nonetheless, it was shocking and upsetting. Each time there is damage, an emotional tax to pay, and scars that accumulate. Following this, some advised me to complain; some advised me not to, saying that complaining may endanger my academic career as an early career researcher. Among those with whom I shared my story—including senior professors who suggested I should make a complaint—no one ever supported me or referred me to any departments that could support me in making my complaint. I did not complain or follow up in any form after all, primarily because I could not afford to do so emotionally and materially at that point.

When I was applying for different vacancies, including PhD positions, I often received a series of responses beginning with phrases like 'I am afraid' or 'I am sorry,' but I often did not hear any further than that, a pitying voice. An unconditional apology often does not work because it does not offer any explanation—all I can say is: 'I apologize.' Or 'I am sorry.' In not saying what I am sorry for, the address fails to reach another (Ahmed, 2013). Thus, it is at best an empty gesture, and at worst, an act of violence through complicity.

As these similar reactions continued repeating themselves over time, I noticed the existence of certain voices of pity for me in almost all of them: voices that lacked any form of empathy. An empathic reaction is one that would be willing to imagine what sort of emotional burden one is going through and what could possibly be done to help. Things do not always go through in an empathic reaction. Empathy is not measured by a checklist, but by how thoroughly an experience has been imagined. In other words, 'empathy is not just remembering to say, that must be really hard; it's figuring out how to bring difficulty into the light so that it can be seen at all' (Jamison, 2011: 4).

Stories of precarious passports are stories of struggles to cross borders and access being denied, and they are emotionally taxing, as much as they are stories of unjust knowledge production and exchange processes. Bathsheba Okwenje puts it very well: manifestations of privilege, precarity, and power should be considered when thinking about any form of collaboration and knowledge exchange across borders and institutions. Struggles of precarious passports reflect the institutionalized and systemic inequalities that develop in our very institutions and can keep reproducing themselves in the absence of any form of truly collective care, systemic empathy, and solidarity. I came to learn how all this could potentially be different thanks to colleagues, employees, fellows, and teachers who truly empathize, care, and take any opportunity to stand in solidarity with colleagues carrying precarious passports, even though they may never have experienced such inequalities themselves. I would hope that imagining a more just path in the academic community would be possible with more solidarity and systemic empathy in practice.

## Acknowledgements

I would like to express my special thanks to Yvette Ruzibiza, Lea Müller-Funk, and Donya Ahmadi for their great and thoughtful responses to the earlier drafts of this piece.

## Works cited

Sara Ahmed, *The Cultural Politics of Emotion* (Routledge, 2013). https://doi.org/10.4324/9780203700372

Sara Ahmed, *Complaint!* (Duke University Press, 2021). https://doi.org/10.1515/9781478022336

Leslie Jamison, *The Empathy Exams: Essays* (Graywolf Press, 2014).

Bathsheba Okwenje, 'Visa applications: Emotional tax and privileged passports', *LSE Blog*, 10 July 2019. https://blogs.lse.ac.uk/africaatlse/2019/07/10/visa-applications-emotional-tax-privileged-passports/

# THE COMPLEXITIES OF PRIVILEGE AND PRECARITY

# 11. Becoming White?

## *Apostolos Andrikopoulos*

Sometime in the mid-1990s, when I was still an elementary school student and lived in a small town in Northern Greece, an old lady told me that dogs were able to recognize Albanians. She insisted it was true. She asked me to stay with her and notice how the neighbor's dog reacted when people passed outside the house. For the time I was there, the dog was quiet and did not react when another Greek neighbor walked in front of the house. At some point, an unknown man appeared in the street and walked along the house's fence. 'An Albanian', the old lady alerted me. The man would have been in his early 20s. His skin was white with red marks from sunburn. He had dark blond curly hair and green eyes. He was wearing a worn-out and oversized pair of trousers and a dirty t-shirt. Suddenly the dog started barking. 'You see?', the old woman asked me. I was astonished. It seemed to me that the woman's claim was confirmed. The dog most likely barked because it saw a stranger, but I did not understand this as a kid. Then the woman provided an explanation for the dog's reaction. According to her, this was due to dogs' instinct to detect thieves and other criminals. The association of Albanians with criminality was rather common and strong at that time. In the 1990s, Albanian migrants were the most stigmatized social group in Greece and were stereotyped as 'delinquents' and 'uncivilized.' These were also the stereotypes for most other migrants in Greece, who predominantly came from the Balkans and countries of the former USSR.

I recently recalled this incident when I was again labeled as a 'white scholar' by a Dutch colleague at the University of Amsterdam. In a Dutch academic context, the category 'white' implies some sort of privilege that our colleagues of color are deprived of. It does not exclusively

    https://doi.org/10.11647/OBP.0331.11

refer to a current privileged position but also to the differentiated access to resources that enable an academic trajectory. The category of 'whiteness' is useful because it allows us to address inequality and the lack of diversity in Dutch academia. But how appropriate is it to apply this category to migrant scholars whose pathway to academia started in contexts in which whiteness had different meanings or was less significant as a marker of privilege?

In my childhood in Greece, whiteness would not self-evidently imply privilege. Those who found themselves at the very margins of society, such as the Albanian man the dog barked for, were white and often had lighter skin colors than those who claimed to be superior to them. This particular meaning of whiteness in Greece, at least in the years I lived there, made me skeptical to accept my categorization as white in the Netherlands. Sometimes I objected to my categorization as such. But then my colleagues (or other interlocutors) would comment that this is another manifestation of my 'white privilege': being able to opt out of a racial categorization. This is something that black people and other people of color cannot easily do. More recently, I came to accept my categorization as 'white', however unenthusiastically, and even used it to describe myself in academic contexts. Nevertheless, I still question the suitability of this category as a means to reflect on my privileges throughout my life and my development as an academic. In this essay, I explore two parallel processes that are somehow interconnected: the first is the shift in my understanding of race throughout my life, from my formative years in Greece up to my recent years in the Netherlands, where I began an academic career as an anthropologist. The second is my own racialization as 'white' since I moved to the Netherlands and became an academic.

I was born and grew up in Kavala, a small provincial city in Northern Greece. Most of Kavala's residents, including my family, were descendants of Greek refugees who were forced to leave their homes in Turkey and settle in Greece. The Treaty of Lausanne (1923), signed after the defeat of Greece in the Greco-Turkish War, obliged Greece and Turkey to exchange populations: Muslim residents of Greece had to migrate to Turkey, and Greek Orthodox residents of Turkey had to move to Greece. The exchange of populations radically changed the demographic composition of Greece. This was especially the case for

Northern Greece, where most refugees settled. Kavala's Muslims, about
half of the total city population, departed for Turkey, and a much greater
number of Greek refugees arrived and settled there. Confronting a
new demographic reality, Greek authorities reoriented their policies
from a model of diversity governance towards a model that prioritized
homogeneity in ethnic and cultural terms.[1]

The dominant narrative until the late 1980s was that Greece had a
highly homogeneous population. Contrary to countries of Western
Europe, which received a considerable number of migrants in the post-
war era, Greece was a country of emigration and, thus, the ethnic profile
of its population was not affected by migration. Despite the presence
of small ethnic, religious, and linguistic minorities in certain regions
of the country, it is not an exaggeration to say that ethnicity and race
were not relevant markers of difference in everyday life. The term racism
(*ratsismos*) was commonly used, but (ironically) rarely in relation to
race (*ratsa*). In that period, the term was mostly used as a synonym for
discrimination on all different grounds (e.g. against children of divorced
parents, homosexual people, or lower-educated people). When I was
born in the early 1980s, inequalities in Kavala were hardly ever related
to ethnicity and race. Only a very small number of residents were non-
Greek or non-white. These were some Roma people and a few Western
Europeans who had come to live in Greece with their Greek spouses.
Also, during the summer months, there were tourists from Germany
and a few other parts of Europe. These are the only encounters I recall
with people of different ethnic and racial backgrounds.

In my primary school, there were no students of non-Greek origin.
I had two classmates whose parents were migrants, but these were
Greek returnees from Germany and Australia. What mattered the most
was the profession of our parents. As there were only public schools

---

1    Interestingly, the first attempt to introduce anthropology in Greek academia
     preceded these events. After the annexation of new lands, including Kavala,
     from the Ottoman Empire (1912–13), Greece faced the challenge of governing
     a very heterogenous population. Seeing how European colonial powers used
     anthropological knowledge in colonial administration, Greece sought expertise
     on the management of diversity within anthropology. Yet the introduction of
     anthropology to university education was eventually abandoned as Greece changed
     approach and adopted a national homogeneity model (Agelopoulos, 2010). It was
     not until the 1980s that anthropology was formally introduced into Greek university
     education.

in the whole region of Kavala, without significant differences in terms of prestige, children from all socio-economic backgrounds studied in the same schools. My classmates whose parents were wealthy and well-educated were usually more articulate, performed better, learned foreign languages, and engaged in extracurricular activities. Many of them continued with a university education, either in Greece or abroad. Not surprisingly, most of these classmates followed professional careers, often similar ones to their parents, and became part of Greece's middle classes.

The composition of the population in Kavala and, more generally, in Greece changed once and for all in the 1990s. As mentioned earlier, Greece used to be a country of emigration, a country from which people left to seek greener pastures elsewhere. Although the country has never been formally colonized,[2] it had an ambiguously subordinate relationship with Europe and more generally with 'the West.' Emigration from Greece to Western Europe was indicative of developmental inequality within Europe and the country's peripheral position. In this constellation of regional and global inequalities, many Greeks developed an admiration for Western Europeans and felt that 'Western' lifestyles and cultural practices were superior and worth imitating (Bakalaki, 2005). But in the 1990s, following the end of the Cold War, Greece became a destination for migrants. These were mostly migrants from former socialist countries of Eastern Europe and the Balkans, undergoing political and economic transformations. The newly settled migrants accounted for almost ten percent of the country's population, and about half were from Albania. For the first time, Greeks came into regular contact in their daily lives with foreigners who were neither tourists nor citizens of wealthier nations. The transformation of Greece into a country of immigration signified for many Greeks that their country had become part of the 'developed world' or, at least, that it was no longer a European periphery. The way Greeks treated migrants and the stereotypes they formed for them directly reflected how they imagined themselves and their country to be in relation to Europe and the world. The projection of migrants as thieves, poor, and uncivilized and the fact that migrants sought a better life in Greece enhanced the self-image of Greeks as resourceful and superior to migrants, and solidified

---

2    However, it has been described as a 'cryptocolony' (Herzfeld, 2002) and more recently as a 'debt-colony'.

the belief that Greece was comparable to countries where Greeks used to migrate to (Andrikopoulos, 2017a; Bakalaki, 2005).

Ethnicity became an important category through which people comprehended social life and everyday interactions. Social class categories became less important than ethnic categories, or were ethnicized. For instance, the derogatory use of the slang term 'kagouras' (a working-class person who unsuccessfully attempts to be fashionable) started being replaced by the term 'Albanian' (e.g. 'What is he wearing today? He really looks like an Albanian'). Similarly, in earlier years, men on the beach whose arms were the only tanned parts of their bodies used to be mocked for having a 'builder's tan' (*maurisma tou oikodomou*). Now, this changed to 'Albanian tan' (*Alvaniko maurisma*). This shift in terms indicates the ethnicization of working classes and the prominent place of migrants in the so-called 3D professions (dirty, difficult, and dangerous). But it also illustrates how difference was inscribed onto the bodies of migrants.

Migrants' bodies became mediums that represented their constructed otherness. Migrants' lives and practices, such as manual work under tough conditions, crafted their bodies in particular ways that rendered them recognizably different (e.g. 'Albanian tan'). But also, the otherness of migrants was often seen to be inherent in their bodies. The old lady in the opening of this essay, for example, believed that criminal behavior is intrinsic in Albanians, and thus, dogs are able to understand it by using their senses. Unlike other contexts, in Greece, this process of racialization was not related to skin color. Nonetheless, this process shared with other cases of racialization that the bodies of migrants came to signify an (assumed) difference and that the essentialization of this difference was used to dehumanize them, subordinate them and exploit them.

In 2001, when I had just started my university education, I worked in a company with more than 100 employees. I worked in the warehouse section, where all my eight colleagues were Albanians. Our employment was not registered, and, as I learned later, it was only us employees at the warehouse who were paid under the table. Despite our work being the most physically intensive, our salaries were the lowest in the company. In addition to this, we had to deal with humiliating and abusive treatment from the owner and director of the company, who came daily to the warehouse to monitor us. Upon entering the warehouse, he started yelling at my colleagues, occasionally at me, for insignificant reasons. Apart from his routine insults and curses, sometimes he became physically violent. Once or twice, he slapped a colleague on his head and kicked another one. On a more regular basis, he threw objects at employees who did not follow his instructions by the letter.

In all these instances, no one protested (including myself). We were all there because we needed income: my colleagues to support their families, myself to support my university education. Once I found a new job, I quit this one. My colleagues stayed in this job for years, and some even referred other family members to work there. On my last day, a Greek colleague from the HR department told me: 'I never understood why you accepted working in the warehouse.' I explained to her that no matter how little the salary was, I was in dire need of money. 'You can do other things. This job is for Albanians,' she replied. Once again, I realized that even if the financial situation of myself and my family was comparable to that of my Albanian colleagues, as a native Greek, I had more opportunities and different access to resources that enabled me to make different decisions. As for my Albanian colleagues, their white skin—which was, in fact, lighter than mine—did not secure them any privilege.

In 2008, at the beginning of the global financial crisis, I moved to the Netherlands, with a full scholarship, to pursue a Master's degree in migration studies. By the time I graduated, Greece had been severely affected by the global financial crisis and faced its own debt crisis. The infamous Troika (International Monetary Fund, Eurogroup, and European Central Bank) offered bailout loans on the premise of reforms and the imposition of severe austerity measures. In these difficult times, the unemployment rate in Greece skyrocketed to almost 30 percent for the general population and reached 60 percent for people of my age. Under this condition, the decision to stay in the Netherlands and try to make a living there was kind of obvious.

In the beginning, I worked as a housekeeper in a hotel. All my colleagues were migrants. Most of them were from the new EU countries in Eastern Europe who had just arrived in the Netherlands and could speak neither Dutch nor English. All of us were paid half of the minimum legal salary (per hour) through a deceptive scheme that made our employer appear legal in the books. I tolerated this situation for several months and left when I found another job. Dutch friends advised me to take legal action against my employer and request to be paid the legal minimum wage, as stipulated in my contract. In addition to the legal process, which concerned only a dispute about my salary, a professor of law, who I had met during my studies, recommended that I report to the Labor Inspectorate that there were violations of the minimum salary for all employees. However, she warned me that if I wanted to do this out of solidarity for my colleagues, I would have to be sure that all of them resided in the Netherlands legally. If the labor inspector went on-site for control and found an unauthorized migrant worker, the worker would be arrested and face the threat of deportation. The EU citizenship of most of my colleagues and me—let alone our white skin—may not have prevented us from working under these exploitative conditions that no other Dutch person had accepted; still, it placed us in a relatively better position than non-EU migrants whose legal status was insecure. Therefore, I had to make sure that my colleagues who were not EU citizens like me resided lawfully in the Netherlands. Only then did I file a complaint. After an entire year of legal processes, which were stressful and time-draining, I only managed to get paid the amount that I should have been paid in the first place. My employer was not fined and did not face any other consequences. Although I testified that all my colleagues were paid under the same terms, the labor inspector was unwilling to investigate the case further. She only asked me if undocumented migrants worked in this hotel. This would have been a solid reason for her to organize an inspection at the worksite, she said. When I replied negatively, she decided to end the case. Years later, once I returned to academia, I came to understand this event in terms of institutional racism.

After the hotel, I started working in the kitchen of a large fast-food restaurant. My colleagues there were also either migrants or migrants' offspring. While I worked at the restaurant, I started applying for PhD positions. After several months of applying for different positions and grants and numerous rejections, an application for a funded PhD position at the University of Amsterdam was successful. My admission into the PhD program of the University of Amsterdam marked the formal beginning of my academic career in the Netherlands and also a new era of relative financial stability. My PhD research was about African migrants in the Netherlands and the new forms of kinship they created, such as through their marriages with Greek and Eastern

European migrants, in a setting of legal exclusion and civic inequality (Andrikopoulos, 2017b). Since many of my colleagues at the restaurant were African migrants and migrants from Europe's periphery, I decided not to quit this job and continued it part-time. My work at the restaurant was no longer a means of earning my living but a form of fieldwork, and a way to meet and network with potential research participants. My colleagues were aware of the reasons I continued working there part-time and many of them became my interlocutors, assisting me in finding other research participants. Looking back I realize how vital my colleagues' assistance was for the success of my research project on an otherwise difficult and sensitive topic.

In the first year of my PhD, I went to Accra, Ghana, to attend a summer school organized by an Ivy League university. Participants in this summer school were mostly US American undergraduate and graduate students, and about a third of them were African Americans. In this summer school, I heard someone referring to me as 'white' for the first time in my life. I shared my surprise with the African American classmate who said it and explained to her why I would not use the term to describe myself. I told her that whiteness had not been a relevant marker of my privileges up to that point in my life and gave her some context about inequalities in Greece and how Albanian migrants came to be racialized as the most significant 'others.' After she listened to me carefully, she asked me whether I thought what I told her was relevant in Ghana and whether I believed that Ghanaians did not think of me as 'white.' Indeed, she had a point.

The same day, we had our first outing as a group in the city. As we walked along a central street in Accra, a few street vendors approached us and tried to sell their stuff. 'Obroni! Obroni!' one of them said to me several times in his effort to attract my attention. I was told that *obroni* means 'white person.' When he realized that I did not intend to buy anything from him, he shifted his attention to others in our group. He approached my African American classmate and addressed her in the same way: 'Obroni! Obroni!' That was a surprise for me. And certainly, for her. In Ghana, people perceive African Americans as *obroni*, the same category they use for white Europeans. Many African Americans who traveled to Ghana as a pilgrimage to the lands of their ancestors were deeply frustrated by this experience (Hartman, 2007). Skin color is not the only criterion for categorizing someone as *obroni* and sometimes skin color and phenotype are irrelevant. Ghanaians call people *obroni* if their mannerisms indicate a privileged position (Darkwah and Adomako Ampofo, 2008). 'We rarely name someone by their appearance as opposed to their character, ability, or trait,' Ghanaian artist Wanlov the Kubolor (2015) maintains and suggests that the term *obroni* originates from the Akan phrase 'abro nipa' meaning 'wicked person.'

In the years that followed, during my PhD and later post-doc, I was classified more and more often as a 'white scholar.' In various academic settings, in the Netherlands and elsewhere, colleagues and students would almost automatically perceive me as 'white.' Sometimes I felt puzzled that I was placed in a category that signified privilege together with scholars whose trajectory to academia had a different point of departure and they had different resources at their disposal. My classification as 'white' prioritized my skin color as a marker of privilege and downplayed its intersection with other characteristics that either enhanced my privileged position—such as me being a man— or undermined it, such as my social class background and origin in Europe's periphery. Perhaps this reflects the predatory capacity of racial categories in the sense that when these notions are strongly loaded, they can gobble other categories of difference with which they intersect. Nevertheless, despite my original discomfort with my classification as 'white,' I gradually came to accept it and became less hesitant to describe myself as such. The reasons for this shift are multiple and interrelated.

As I became more and more part of the society I was living in, I had to relate with categories of difference that were meaningful there. Now I live in a society where social inequalities are racialized. These inequalities are visibly clear when I walk out of my university campus. I encounter more people of different ethnic and racial backgrounds in the city than among my students and colleagues (see Wekker et al., 2016). Moreover, as an anthropologist who has conducted research on racialized African migrants in Europe, the category of 'white' is useful for reflecting on my positionality in relation to my interlocutors and the privileges my academic position entails. Nevertheless, this does not mean that African migrants in the Netherlands place me in the same category with white Dutch. A finding of my PhD research was that African migrant men who got a residence permit through marriage preferred a spouse from Europe's periphery, such as Greece or Poland, than a white Dutch woman. They were concerned that their legalization through marriage would place them in a highly unequal position in the relationship and make them dependent on their spouses. Thus, they preferred women who were more or less in a similar socio-economic position, such as working-class migrants from Europe's periphery, for whom they could also care in material terms. For my African interlocutors in the Netherlands, I was undoubtedly white but not as white as native Dutch people.

As I continued my academic career and climbed a few steps in the academic hierarchy, I became more similar in terms of privileges to my Dutch colleagues and more different than my colleagues in Greece. Even as a PhD student in the Netherlands, my salary was comparable to the salary of an Associate Professor in Greece and, furthermore, I had access to resources that allowed me to make my work more widely known and therefore less marginal in academic debates of my field. These are important reasons that might explain how I came to use the term 'white' as a means to reflect on my current privileges. But does this mean that I became white? This is a question that I have yet to answer.

# Acknowledgements

I would like to thank Ladan Rahbari and Olga Burlyuk for their invitation to participate in this collection and their attentive reading of my essay. I am also grateful to Myriam Lamrani and Joël Illidge for their comments on an earlier version of the manuscript. I acknowledge that I wrote this essay during a Marie Skłodowska-Curie fellowship which was funded from the EU's Horizon 2020 research and innovation programme under the grant agreement No 894547.

# Works cited

Georgios Agelopoulos, 'Contested territories and the quest for ethnology: People and places in Izmir 1919–1922', in *Spatial Conceptions of the Nation: Modernizing Geographies in Greece and Turkey*, edited by N. Diamantouros, T. Dragonas, and C. Keyder (Bloomsbury Publishing, 2010), pp. 181–191.

Apostolos Andrikopoulos, 'Hospitality and immigration in a Greek urban neighborhood: An ethnography of mimesis', *City & Society*, 29/2 (2017a): 281–304. https://doi.org/10.1111/ciso.12127

Apostolos Andrikopoulos, Argonauts of West Africa: Migration, citizenship and kinship dynamics in a changing Europe, PhD dissertation (University of Amsterdam, 2017b).

Alexandra Bakalaki, 'L'envie, moteur de l'imitation,' *Ethnologie Française*, 35/2 (2005): 317–327. https://doi.org/10.3917/ethn.052.0317

Akosua Darkwah and Ampofo Adomako, 'Race, gender and global love: Non-Ghanaian wives, insiders or outsiders in Ghana?' *International Journal of Sociology of the Family* (2008): 187–208.

Saidiya Hartman, *Lose Your Mother: A Journey Along the Atlantic Slave Route* (Farrar, Straus and Giroux, 2007).

Michael Herzfeld, 'The absence presence: Discourses of crypto-colonialism', *The South Atlantic Quarterly* 101/4 (2002): 899–926. https://doi.org/10.1215/00382876-101-4-899

Wanlov the Kubolor, 'Obroni, a history,' *Africa is a Country* (2015). https://africasacountry.com/2015/03/whitehistorymonth-obroni-a-history

Gloria Wekker, Rosalba Icaza, Hans Jansen, Marieke Slootman, and Rolando Vázquez, *Let's Do Diversity: Report of the Diversity Commission, University of Amsterdam* (University of Amsterdam, 2016).

# 12. Academic Mobility the 'Other' Way: Embodying Simultaneous Privilege and Precarity

*Karolina Kluczewska*

Usually, international academic mobility is about moving from the non-West to the West or closer to the West, and rarely the 'other' way round. I grew up in Poland, in between the West and non-West, and went both ways. The truly transformative episode of academic mobility was related to my integration experience in the non-West, specifically in Tajik academia. There, my identity and interiorized academic practices and standards were questioned, making me rethink my positionality and reflect on the simultaneous conditions of privilege and precarity.

I moved abroad from Poland right after high school and relatively easily learned to navigate various academic cultures. I did my Bachelor's degree in Italy, with an Erasmus exchange in Germany. Then, I received my Master's degree in the United Kingdom. After that, I worked in the development sector in Tajikistan for two years before going back to the United Kingdom for a PhD program. Given that my research was about the development aid scene in Tajikistan, I returned there and became affiliated with a local university while doing fieldwork. After the PhD my academic mobility only intensified, which is the common story of most graduates who stubbornly stick to research on niche topics or related to regions without a strategic geopolitical significance, and consequently struggle to find a stable research position. Thus, I embarked on a post-doctoral fellowship in France, simultaneously obtained a research

 https://doi.org/10.11647/OBP.0331.12

and teaching position in Russia, followed by fellowships and teaching assignments at three German universities. Later, I moved to Belgium.

Over several years, while working at various Western universities, I did regular fieldwork in Tajikistan and remained affiliated with a local university there. This essay is a reflection on my cumulative stay in Tajik academia, which included several stays ranging from two to fourteen months at a time. I did not really struggle as a student (or, later, as a researcher) in Western academia. Yes, initially, when I moved to the United Kingdom for my MA studies, I was surprised that we had to write so many essays, while most of my previous exams in Italy had been oral. But that was really the only noticeable difference. I am, after all, a product of Western academia when it comes to the conventions of doing research, publishing, and teaching—all of which, despite unarguable differences between individual countries, follow similar rules throughout the West.

Going from my home country towards the East was more challenging. This was particularly the case when trying to navigate the hermetic and impoverished academia in Tajikistan, a country that is notoriously described as the poorest in the former Soviet Union. An affiliation with one of the Tajik universities secured my research visa and exposed me to academic cultures operating according to criteria that were new to me. From my undeniably Eurocentric point of view, they sometimes seemed to contradict common sense. Experiences of building relations with university staff and local colleagues, new types of relationality, and new research and teaching standards taught me about Tajik academia. Moreover, all this offered a fresh lens to view where I came from as an academic.

## Why are you here?

My integration into Tajik academia is not the story of an outsider who received preferential treatment solely because of white color, Western university affiliation, and an EU passport in her pocket. In terms of relationships between foreign academics and locals, Tajik academia can be seen as a truly decolonial place—with its own ways of knowing and doing. It forces outsiders to do their best so that their presence can be locally perceived as legitimate and welcome. The main task is not to build trust from zero: first, you need to eliminate the underlying distrust to get to the zero starting point.

I cannot think of one interaction with new local colleagues that did not start with curiosity (and even astonishment) on their side as to why I was there. Often, this was just genuine disbelief about why someone from Europe would be willing to spend time at a Tajik university. In some cases, however, curiosity was accompanied by suspicion about the *real* reason for my stay in the country (other than research) or the *actual* topic of my interest (other than development aid).

This attitude was not directed towards me personally and needs to be placed in a broader context. The first underlying reason is the legacy of Soviet-era attitudes to foreigners. Suspicion towards people coming from the Western bloc was an outcome of the isolationist policies of the Soviet Union and the paranoid attitudes of Soviet security services involved in the surveillance of foreigners. Moreover, Tajik academia is a place of emigration, not immigration. Since the country's independence from the Soviet Union in 1991, local universities and research institutes have constantly witnessed mass emigration of skilled cadres. Consequently, when so many academics want to learn English and attempt to go to Russia or further West, it appears logical to question why someone would learn Tajik and go against the tide. While some foreign scholars stayed in the country in the 1990s, during the civil war (1992–1997) and in its aftermath, the number of foreign researchers regularly coming to Tajikistan could literally be counted on the fingers of two hands, and the number of those periodically staying at Tajik research institutions on one hand. As a result, for many local colleagues, I was the first researcher coming from the West whom they had seen in university corridors and classrooms for a prolonged time. Finally, my positionality might be confusing: I grew up in Poland but had lived in several other countries, so where did I actually come from? And, if I 'had made it' from a post-communist country to the West, why did I come to Tajikistan?

In practice, the suspicion manifested itself in administrative obstacles that were artificially created. For example, an extraordinary amount of additional supporting documents was requested for my background check. For the same reason, in order to become more visible, I became actively involved in university life through teaching, assisting with organizing conferences, and giving presentations. As one colleague told me: 'Everyone needs to see what you are doing all the time.' Although time-consuming and distracting from my actual research, my activities at the university resulted in intensifying and improving my relations with local scholars.

One extreme case of distrust concerned an employee who suggested to several colleagues that I might be a spy. The position of power that this person occupied implied that their personal attitude could have serious implications for my reputation and my stay in the country. When I first heard about their suspicion towards me, I lost my composure and cried aloud in a university corridor because of the sense of injustice. At that moment, I thought that my only fault was that I truly liked the place, learned the language, and wanted to build meaningful relations with local researchers, which happened to look suspicious in a place that so many wanted to leave.

Later, I realized that my fault was that I was part of the unjust global economic system, and I found myself at the intersection of Western and non-Western academia. When the two clashed, a blinking red 'error' sign came on. I could be an average early-career academic in the West, struggling with the pressure to publish, constantly preparing job applications, and navigating short-term contracts, which required me to move between cities and countries. Yet for scholars in Tajikistan, I looked so privileged that I could not avoid suspicion. In Tajikistan, PhD students and early-career researchers do not apply for research and travel grants to go to a different continent a few times per year because there is no national research foundation nor university funds where they could apply for such funding. Local academics could rightfully wonder who would pay for a PhD student's frequent flights to Tajikistan when one return ticket, say, Paris-Dushanbe, costs the equivalent of the three-month salary of a local university professor. And how can a 20-something-year-old girl move from one Western European country to another each year, when established local scholars cannot afford to go to a neighboring country for a conference?

The Tajik academic environment clearly differs from Western academia, which promotes internationalization by facilitating foreign student and staff recruitment. Precisely because of its openly hermetic nature, it appears more honest than Western academia, which prides itself on transparency and meritocracy, yet we all know that what often helps to secure jobs are personal connections and informal recommendations. There are walls to climb to integrate into these two environments. These walls in Tajik academia are thick and made of bricks, and you see them from the start. In Western academia, these walls are made of glass, and so you might not notice them at first glimpse—but they are still there.

## One good turn deserves another

Tajik academia has also exposed me to a new type of relationality in the way people are connected in an academic setting and in society more broadly. The practice of mutual favors is locally called *khizmat*, which literally translates as a service and implies that this is a service that solves problems. *Khizmat* is an intrinsic part of Tajik academia because it complements existing rules which, on their own, do not allow for the effective functioning of universities. It is an informal institution of exchange and support, which allows for advancing careers, avoiding bureaucracy, and distributing big workloads. *Khizmat* involves a social obligation: favors done by one person translate into the long-term loyalty, gratitude, and indebtedness of the other. Because it results in the long-term subordination of the person who was granted the favor, *khizmat* can be seen as a form of patron-client relationship. This practice relies on existing social and professional hierarchies and, at the same time, reproduces them. Favors that have a low cost for those who do them can mean the world for those who receive them.

Sometimes, *khizmat* can happen when you least expect it. The problem with the university staff member in a position of power, who insinuated that I might be a spy rather than simply a researcher going the 'other' way, was resolved accidentally through a *khizmat*. Because of this artificially created conundrum at the university, my spirits were rather low in those days. One of my neighbors noticed this. I was on good terms with this person, and they were also an influential person in society. When I explained the problem I was facing, my neighbor asked about that staff member's name, and then swore really loudly. It turned out that my neighbor not only knew the person, but also had done them a favor several years ago. My neighbor took out their mobile phone and called that staff member. When this person answered, the two exchanged conventional, cordial greetings, asking about health, how families were doing and how work was going. After that, the conversation continued nonchalantly:

> My neighbor: Please do not bother my *shogird* (student, protégée).
>
> The other person: Who is your *shogird*?
>
> My neighbor: Karolina, she is my *shogird*. I took care of her, I helped her when she moved here, I found her a job, I taught her Tajik.

My relationship with the neighbor did not actually go nearly that far. This is, however, how *khizmat* works. To convince the university staff member, my neighbor did not refer to objective facts (such as, hypothetically, me being a polite neighbor or me speaking the language). Instead, they used the argument that I was being protected by them. According to this logic, what mattered was that if this person bothered me, they also bothered my neighbor. My neighbor's words had an immediate effect, as all problems at the university ceased immediately. At the same time, I became indebted to my neighbor. One good turn deserves another. Soon, I started repaying the favor by writing and translating texts related to my neighbor's job.

Nevertheless, I was still a privileged researcher from Western academia, with all flights and other fieldwork expenses covered. In Tajik academia, in turn, the combination of factors such as gender (female), age (mid- to late 20s), status (PhD student and then a post-doctoral fellow), and origin (unclear, but in any case, foreign) placed me at the subordinate end of the *khizmat* system. Those who are at its upper end are usually, although not exclusively, male, middle-aged professors from influential local families. With my positionality, one cannot say no to requests from different sides because there is a lot at stake. One phone call can resolve your problems and can also create them.

My relationships with peers have always been good: balanced, supportive, and intellectually stimulating. However, through various forms of *khizmat* I became indebted to many senior colleagues—literally, although not financially. As a result, *khizmat*-related obligations kept me busy and nervous. I did some editing or translated presentations for upcoming conferences. I took over some classes for one colleague, *ad hoc*. Sometimes this person informed me about 'my' class one hour before it was supposed to take place, on the other side of the city. At times, I did not even know what topic it was supposed to be about.

Rather than a never-ending cycle of indebtedness, such deeds are usually presented as an honor for a *shogird*, a reason to be proud because you can support respected scholars. The *khizmat* system sustains itself because relations with colleagues are simultaneously personal and professional: they mix personal characteristics with institutional prerogatives. It is not solely a system based on exploitation: the patron's personal reputation is your guarantee.

*Khizmat* can be excessive and tends to be used to exaggeration. Importantly, it is not only a feature of Tajik academia. Several similar practices exist in Western academia, although they are framed more subtly. Networking at academic events, a widely encouraged practice, often involves scanning participant lists to identify the ones who can facilitate one's career. In some Western countries, PhD students refer to their supervisors as 'doctoral fathers/mothers,' which implies a personalized, subordinated relationship. Then, we hear stories about established scholars who simply add their names to publications entirely written by junior researchers seeking to publish for the first time. So is Western academia really that different?

## No need to do more

Another formative experience I owe to Tajik academia is exposure to the culture of mediocracy. This is an approach that sets the standards of academic life, such as studying and reasoning. As the name suggests, mediocrity at university is preferred. As a student, teacher, and researcher, you need to do certain things—study, teach, and research. While you should fulfil the minimum criteria, you do not have to aspire to be better than average. It is enough to do just enough.

The culture of mediocracy is the opposite of the culture of excellence, which guides studying, teaching, and research in the West. The obsession with striving for excellence manifests itself in often-used keywords indicating constant, linear development: 'feedback,' 'progress,' and 'intellectual growth.' It is visible in the importance of guidance criteria and corresponding assessment systems, such as several university rankings and league tables helping students choose the best degree, the *Exzellenzinitiative* in Germany and the Research Excellence Framework (REF) in the United Kingdom, or the recent Teaching Excellence and Student Outcomes Framework (TEF) introduced in England. This is not to say that Western academia *is* excellent. Rather, it approaches excellence through the prism of one-size-fits-all quantitative metrics.

In Tajik academia, in contrast, the performance standards (for example, good, average, and bad) are set not according to some pre-established criteria. Instead, they are established on a contextual basis. This occurs by taking one person who is worse than others and one who is better than others in a given group, and treating them as referral points of bad and good performance, respectively. The best position is the one in-between. In Tajikistan, it is socially expected to be like others and not stand out from the crowd. There is also a strong underlying economic component of the culture of mediocrity.

This approach underlies academic practices, and it is accompanied by a high degree of performativity, and even theatricality. For example, academic events which I attended often involved elevated discussions on issues such as orthography, grammar mistakes, and inconsistent referencing styles, rather than focusing on the content of the texts that were presented.

Besides some observations concerning research practices, I mostly became familiar with the culture of mediocrity in my classroom, when interacting with students. It started from the issue of attendance. While attending classes was mandatory, usually only seven or eight students were present in a class of about 15. When some professors complained about the low attendance rate, all students would come to classes for the next few days, and then everything would go back to how it usually was. Out of the eight attending students, only half would come punctually, and the rest would appear gradually throughout the class. Once everyone was in the classroom, a few students would start asking to be allowed to leave earlier, most often for the following reasons: 'There is no one at home and I need to take care of younger siblings'; 'I have an appointment with local authorities'; or 'I need to take a bus before the peak time.' To be a mediocre student, it is important to attend classes from time to time in order not to be expelled from the university, and you are also expected to sporadically say something during the class. Only one or two students in each group actively participated in classes.

Then, there was the issue of student essays and plagiarism. Once I visited an internet café near my house to print out some documents. A long queue of students was waiting at the counter. The café's employee noticed that I was older and kindly apologized: 'You need to wait a bit, they are printing their essays.' While waiting, I realized that actually the students were not printing *their* essays, but pre-written essays. There was an impressive collection of model essays on standard questions assigned in various faculties, from biology to linguistics, in the file stored on the main computer. The students were simply spelling their names to the café's employees, who typed them on cover pages with various logos, depending on the local university they attended. If some topics were missing, the employee would quickly download them from the internet. Again, to be a mediocre student, it is important to hand in a good essay—but it does not need to be written by you.

From my Eurocentric point of view, for a long time, this seemed illogical. While it is prestigious to be a student in Tajikistan, what is the point of studying if it resembles a Potemkin village? Then, I realized that probably there is indeed no point in doing more, striving for excellence, if you know from the start that there will be no reward for your efforts. Of nine million Tajik citizens, 1.5 are labor migrants in Russia, working in the construction and service sectors. These are not only low-skilled migrants, but often people with university degrees, too. The only sector that pays well in the country is international development, which is already saturated. The priority, anyway, is given to graduates with a university degree from the West. In turn, working for government agencies at entry-level positions does not allow you to sustain yourself, let alone your family, and to land a well-paid job, you need connections. Seen in this light, indeed, why bother? It is laudable that some students still do not give up trying in the face of their gloomy career prospects.

The illumination occurred slowly, through different scenarios, such as when, one day just after my class finished, I met a good colleague. I praised one of the students, saying how dedicated the young man was.

Karolina: He has a bright future ahead of him!

My colleague: No, others have a bright future. He doesn't.

My colleague was clearly amused at my logic. Seeing my reaction, they explained: 'They have someone else to make their future bright. He doesn't.' Academic work is not much different. While it is prestigious to be a student, there is little prestige associated with working at the university because of the low salaries. Many of my colleagues continued working in academia only because they liked it, not because of incentives related to salaries or career growth. Others continued because of a lack of other options. They had little time to prepare for their classes because they usually taught for several hours per day. Consequently, sometimes their preparation was limited to glancing over Wikipedia pages or dictating to the students some recycled sentences related to course topics. Young female lecturers, in particular, struggled with problematic student behavior, as well as the household chores and childcare that awaited them at home. Naturally, the quality of their teaching and publications suffered as a result.

Encounters with the culture of mediocracy allowed me to see the culture of excellence of Western academia from a new perspective. On the one hand, it is such a privilege to strive for excellence when one has a decent living and rewards are visible on the horizon. On the other hand, the cost of the excellence culture combined with the precarity inscribed in Western academia is high. Students feel that they need to have the best grades and do several internships to increase their chances of obtaining a good job in a job market flooded with highly qualified graduates. Often, they also worry about the debts they have accumulated during university years, given that in several countries annual student fees amount to thousands or even tens of thousands of euros, dollars, or pounds. Early-career researchers, in turn, feel a pressure to publish (a lot and in good journals) and are forced to compete with friends for the same, scarce (and often not really attractive) positions. Just because we do not want to remain jobless, after all our efforts so far.

In both cases, there are structural obstacles. Students and scholars in Tajikistan have few incentives to be more than mediocre. In Western academia, in turn, we feel pressured to constantly perform above the average, and aspire to excellence defined by strict criteria of performance indicators, impact factors, and other types of metrics.

# The story continues

This is only one story about integrating into Tajik academia as a foreign researcher, and there are so many other stories to be told about it. In Tajik academia, I met so many interesting colleagues, and learned from them, as scholars and humans. I enjoyed refreshing conversations with students and felt inspired by their unique views on life and world politics. This academic environment is not devoid of challenges, but it also has many positive sides, such as the lack of a rat race and absence of quantitative metrics and performance standards. Moreover, as a researcher coming from the West, I found going the 'other' way transformative. Searching for my place in Tajik academia convinced me that positionality is both about how we see ourselves and how others see us. Our characteristics—such as gender, age, status, and origin—overlap with local frames and can function as double-edged swords, depending on the situation. Navigating Tajik academia showed me that precarity and privilege are two sides of the same coin. You can be a precarious and a privileged researcher simultaneously, depending on which of the various academic cultures you belong to is the reference point.

As I write this essay, I am again in a new place—this time in Belgium, exploring a new academic landscape. This is what academia looks like nowadays: migrant academics are constantly on the move. Stories of academic mobility are stories with no clear beginning and no clear ending. We carry our multiple belongings, mixed identities, and complex positionalities from university to university, from country to country, and reshape ourselves, again and again.

# 13. 'A Small Plot of New Land at All Times': A Narrative of a Vulnerability Mortified

## *Bojan Savić*

This is how it should be done: Lodge yourself on a stratum, experiment with the opportunities it offers, find an advantageous place on it, find potential movements of deterritorialization, possible lines of flight, experience them, produce flow conjunctions here and there, try out continuums of intensities segment by segment, have a small plot of new land at all times.

Deleuze and Guattari, *A Thousand Plateaus* (2013), p. 161.

Perhaps my zeal for places and geographies different from those of my childhood and adolescence can explain why I have rarely experienced life beyond the reassuring promise of progress. My thirst to go and be somewhere else, to move ostensibly forward, has somehow always been quenched. That has probably allowed me to disregard questions about the personal cost, toil, or unsteadiness of the forward motion—or the cost of choosing academia as the vehicle for it. Clearly, I have only ever lived my own life, but I have witnessed the denial of one's own vulnerability in many of my colleagues. I have not researched this frail subjectivity enough to say anything of broader value, but I can poke and prod my own formation as a forward-looking scholarly ascetic and my reflection may resonate with the reader. So, iterative spatial movement toward the Other as a bulwark against felt risk and instability—a paradox and a strange little equation.

It was not until years after I had left Belgrade to study and live abroad that I realized the 'where' of why my life had always been about

    https://doi.org/10.11647/OBP.0331.13

finding 'a small plot of new land at all times' (Deleuze and Guattari, 2013, 161); moving from places I had methodically molded into homes, only to find new spaces and create new hearths. And leave them again. Looking back at years of fretful motion and geographic angst, I have lived in dislocated space over two decades of both joyful and sorrowful deterritorialization and reterritorialization (Deleuze and Guattari, 2013). Skeptical of localism and the 'poetics of place' (Prieto, 2012), I have likewise resented their patronizing rejections (e.g., 'cosmopolitanism'). Instead, I have found myself viscerally in love with space *as spacing*, with space as a distancing motion rather than a finite expanse. Perhaps that is because every motion of dissociation has set me up for new proximities. Each spacing has come with new routines; with every distance I have sought new familiarity. I have fortified my love for social space through its critique rather than, say, bittersweet wanderlust. In fact, I have nourished this love through Other spaces, Other struggles, and Other aesthetics. At once consumed by seeing antagonisms everywhere and enchanted with spatial difference, I have pursued homes through unmooring and dislocation.

That has been my experience of space. And what of my time? Clearly, time is in the passage of difference, in the reversals and disruptions of movement across beloved towns and rooms, in the intimate upheavals of abandoned and treasured familiarities. I have come to understand my intimate spatiality as a sentimental 'line of flight' (Deleuze and Guattari, 2013), an unrelenting possibility of makeovers. Sutured into it, my temporality has been a never-ending event of change, aspiration, and hope.

Moreover, for as long as I can remember, I have only known how to hope, at times hoping against hope, as the famous Pauline maxim goes. Defeats have had to be merely transient trials, and humiliations have been calls to step up to the plate and defend what has always been dearest to me—work, the sheer physics of effort. I have seen none of this as particularly virtuous, related to ethics, or even as useful or 'smart'. Instead, my emotional investments in hope and work have merely been the facts of my identity, habits that have made me feel anchored, even when I understood little about myself or the social world around me—as a preschool boy, a teenager, or more recently as an adult. Either way, the ecstasy of labor has outshone all, including eating popcorn or really nothing for dinner, impossible financial choices, being called 'Serbian' where being Serbian was scarcely a good thing, being called 'pretty white for a Syrian' (oh, the layers of irony), enduring casual toxicity because sleeping on the street would have been worse, etc. The will to improve compelled me to see tests (more so than 'difficulties') as mere mechanics of life, stripped of any need for deeper reflection, immersion, affect, or even memory. Moreover, I ignored my loved ones' own memories and accounts of my experiences that could have easily felt like pain and vulnerability.

Creating a home, tearing it down, and reinventing intimacy elsewhere, in a new place of trials, meant so much only because it was part of this labor and physicality. I had no time or patience for my own story while I was pushing myself to seek out the stories of Others. Seeing Others in the way I never even considered I would need to see myself was exhilarating. In that gaze, I found the same force that had propelled my deterritorialization. In other words, the interest I felt for the Other stood alongside the hope I felt for my lifepath. And yet, it took me years to connect the dots and begin to understand myself the way I had worked to understand Others; years to carve out a liminal space and become my Other. Not only did I have to move towns, countries, houses, and continents; I had to deterritorialize and displace my sense of merit and normality and re-envision my life and body as *perhaps* subject to wider relations of power—classed, raced, sexed, or otherwise.

Writing and rereading this, I return to a question that has troubled me for years. What does my neglect of my own experiences of vulnerability as a junior working-class academic from the European periphery convey? It feels like an intimate genealogy of something I have recognized while living and working *elsewhere*—in Western Afghanistan, Eastern Poland, small-town North Carolina, Istanbul's gentrifying neighborhoods, Virginian DC suburbs, the post-colonial immigrant neighborhoods of Brussels, my native Serbia, etc. But I still cannot quite define it. While I cannot think them apart, I also cannot grasp my subjectivity of hope and work in relation to my disregard for the possibility of personal precarity. Is my conundrum an expression of capitalist 'personal responsibility' or am I articulating a proletarian 'master of self' ethics (Polanyi, 2018, 20), especially given my research interest in the post-colonial politics of vulnerability? Where do my investments in 'work' and 'hope' belong?

I am skeptical of both 'capitalist' and 'proletarian' ethics as drivers of my desires, especially since I cannot quite frame my familial childhood space, my family friends and close relatives, or the school environment in terms of either. After all, my research interests animate my passion for academia, and they have shifted, teetered, and morphed over time, so why would my values remain stable or even entirely clear? Moreover, how 'proletarian' is it to be oblivious to personal vulnerability? If anything, I sound like a regrettable example of Engels' musings on 'false (class) consciousness' (Eagleton, 1994). I remember once believing in merit as a personal code of conduct, but even then (over a decade ago), I never associated it with social order or a philosophy of ethics. I have always seen my investment in work as just about the only strategy available to me, the only tool I (have) had to gratify my compulsion for movement.

It would be easy, then, to say that I have never quite thought of myself as a vulnerable subject because I have always inhabited a space-time of aspirant movement or because I have been stirred by some inner compulsion, a fire to keep finding new places that will feel like an old home. 'You're a dreamer,' my paternal grandma once told me, only to contrast that with a heartfelt recommendation to 'instead, become a priest' and 'put dreams to good use.' All this would be a neat little summary of the life of an academic who has moved between something that is gently called 'multiple Europes' (Whitehead et al., 2019) of ethnic, linguistic, artistic, religious, class, and political diversities and something else decried as 'American hegemony' (Agnew, 2005). This neat account would not be altogether wrong. I have indeed spent years casually mortifying any thoughts or confessions of personal vulnerability in favor of an intense subjectivity of pursuit and hope. But each of my quests for 'a small plot of new land' drew up new boundaries, separating me from the familiar, from the beloved and unloved. Each unmooring and berthing edified a Self attached to lonely and elusive attempts to understand the vulnerabilities of Others. Of Others—meaning not of myself.

Therefore, I want to reframe the ethical dichotomy I have mentioned above. More than an internalized struggle of capitalist and proletarian ethics, or the pursuit of movement to 'keep busy,' my aspirational asceticism and its mortification of a different socioeconomic subjectivity has more chaotic sources. It is also a very bodily sentiment cultivated through parental care, a device that has enabled me to endure long waits for job, scholarship, and graduate school interviews, empty fridges, uncertain funding or employment contract renewals, worn-out mattresses, and an unrelenting sense of relative deprivation that haunted me for years from Belgrade to Maastricht, Istanbul, and elsewhere across Europe and the United States. (It is hilariously strange to be so privileged to experience crippling want in so many different corners of the world.) Since parental care has partially underwritten my aspirational experience of time and space, I have always appreciated hope as an artefact of my parents' love and have, therefore, always clung to it. Beyond that, hoping against hope has at times been a galvanizing force that has yielded exactly that which I needed desperately—the ability to 'pick myself up off the floor.' No other fuel, no other nudge. Just the redemptive work of inner compulsion.

Finally, I was born (and grew up) in a place that seemed unconcerned with what others have described as 'self-love' (Knox, 2018; Neuhouser, 2008; Force, 1997) and 'self-care' (Squire and Nicolazzo, 2019; Michaeli, 2017), or attitudes attributed to mixtures of religious, economic, political, familial, and other social ethics. Growing up, I was conditioned to see any purposeful focus on self (and particularly Self) as narcissism, egocentricity, and greed. In an environment of protracted political and socioeconomic collapse during the long 1990s, the familial and communal sharing of food, stories, clothes, emotions, and housing were matters of survival across the former Yugoslavia. Therefore, any centering of self (unless it came from pop-culture celebrities) used to cause something of bewilderment. In my family, it felt vaguely inappropriate and, to me, in that context, it seemed unthinkable. Not so much explicitly undesirable (although I may have felt that as well), but aporetic (Derrida, 1993). To seek good for Self, to care for Self as distinct from the Other felt impossible in the sense of being self-defeating, illogical, and personally unhelpful. For the Other (the neighbor, the relative, the workplace supervisor, etc.) was one's own best guarantee for survival. To sideline mutual reliance in favor of Self and 'independence' seemed foolhardy. (And yet, the more privileged Other did just that routinely.) Once, after my dad's impatience with a nosy neighbor resulted in a minor squabble between them, my mom called his attitude 'abnormal'. (Yes, Serbian expressions may sound odd to a foreign ear.) 'We need everyone,' she said. 'So what if they stop by our apartment unannounced and ask what I cooked for lunch? Who cares?' I vigorously agreed with my mom. It did not occur to me to think that our lives were so precarious that we could not even afford privacy. A decade later, in college, I intuitively understood private/public and inside/outside hierarchies as boundaries of power and as particularly bourgeois values, privileges, and spacings (Ellison, 1983; Arendt, 1961). Therefore, juxtaposed with the ethics of self-elision as a prudent strategy for survival that was only ostensibly paradoxical, self-care and self-centered thought seemed superfluous, rude, and even self-destructive. It was an attitude I took for granted, much like the sentiments of hope my parents instilled in me. Coupled with a life of scholarly wariness of capitalism, communism, and other 'metanarratives,' such circumstances conditioned me to readily ignore any need to situate myself where I have embedded everything else—in pervasive and permeating relations of power.

Therefore, when I speak about space-as-spacing, about my various journeys, and my vulnerabilities, I speak of them in terms of dislocation. They can be merely deterritorialized and reterritorialized rather than alleviated or improved. I can only mortify their unsettling effects; not deny or erase them but continue to move them around so that they can yield new sites and moments of hope.

I apologize to the reader if my correlation of dislocation, aspiration, work, and vulnerability is less than clear. It is not as straightforward as saying 'I have to keep working so that I can afford to keep moving; therefore, I have no time to think about precarity,' but it also need not be as convoluted as this text suggests. Dislocation, aspiration, work, and precarity are correlated in my inability to think about them separately. They are correlated in my awareness that my life of academic asceticism and nomadism is a precarious one, but one beyond which I do not exist, because beyond it, I have nothing conceivable to aspire to. Perhaps the bond between dislocation and work that I have been trying to describe is akin to what Charteris, Nye, and Jones (2017) refer to as the 'scope for freedom' (ibid., 53), as resistance to the elusive space of 'the academy' (ibid., 49–64) and to the underpaid and precarious work it offers its members.

# Works cited

John Agnew, *Hegemony: The New Shape of Global Power* (Temple University Press, 2007).

Hannah Arendt and Jerome Kohn, *Between Past and Future* (Penguin, 2006).

Jennifer Charteris, Adele Nye, and Marguerite Jones, *Wild Choreography of Affect and Ecstasy: Contentious Pleasure (Joussiance) in the Academy* (Brill, 2017). https://brill.com/view/book/edcoll/9789463511797/BP000006.xml

Gilles Deleuze and Félix Guattari, *A Thousand Plateaus: Capitalism and Schizophrenia* (Bloomsbury Academic, 2013).

Jacques Derrida, *Aporias*, translated by Thomas Dutoit (Stanford University Press, 1993).

Dian Squire and Z. Nicolazzo, 'Love my naps, but stay woke: The case against self-care,' *About Campus* 24/2 (2019): 4–11. https://doi.org/10.1177/1086482219869997

Terry Eagleton, *Ideology* (Routledge, 1994).

Charles Ellison, 'Marx and the modern city: Public life and the problem of personality,' *The Review of Politics* 45/3 (1983): 393–420. https://doi.org/10.1017/S0034670500044855

Pierre Force, 'Self-love, identification, and the origin of political economy,' *Yale French Studies*, 92 (1997): 46–64. https://doi.org/10.2307/2930386

Andy Knox, 'Examining self-love, love of the 'other' and love of the 'enemy': A reply to Mitchell,' *Global Discourse* 8/4 (2018): 610–614. https://doi.org/10.1080/23269995.2018.1530917

Inna Michaeli, 'Self-care: An act of political warfare or a neoliberal trap?' *Development* 60/1 (2017): 50–56. https://doi.org/10.1057/s41301-017-0131-8

Frederick Neuhouser, *Rousseau's Theodicy of Self-Love: Evil, Rationality, and the Drive for Recognition* (Oxford University Press, 2008).

Karl Polanyi, *Economy and Society: Selected Writings* (John Wiley & Sons, 2018).

Eric Prieto, *Literature, Geography, and the Postmodern Poetics of Place* (Palgrave Macmillan, 2012).

Christopher Whitehead, Susannah Eckersley, Mads Daugbjerg, and Gönül Bozoğlu, *Dimensions of Heritage and Memory: Multiple Europes and the Politics of Crisis* (Routledge, 2019). https://doi.org/10.4324/9781138589476

# 14. Conversation with San Precario

*Alexander Strelkov*

O, San Precario, protector of the humble multitude,

You watch over all of us, irrespective of color, creed, ethno-cultural background and the like. To all trades and occupations that face misery, near-certain demise, and precarity in all its possible forms do you grant your benediction. You give hope to all of us, from those toiling in the Bangladeshi sweatshops, call centers and chain stores to academic nomads, who are driven ever further by the destruction of the tenure habitat like the poor orangutan on Borneo. Let me converse with you, I beseech, share the burden of my heart and give your guidance in these tumultuous times. Swirling in the sea of precarity, more than ten years ago I set sail into the unknown, hoping to reach the promised land of academic excellence and analytical zeal.

Though small, my vessel was not without rigging and gear. Master NK trained me, as well and as diligently as a diamond cutter from Antwerp polishes his/her wares to be sold at Gassan's in Amsterdam. Yet when I think of it now, has he trained me too well, instilled in me some weird creed of professional responsibility? For years later I would be asked to not have hour-long meetings with undergrads in a common office, explaining to them the intricacies of the social science trade. Moreover, I could sweet talk the customs officer, for he tried to deprive me of books on EU integration, which I duly cherished. Lucky was I, for my parents supported me, and the benevolent staff of Max-Planck-Institüt für Gesellschaftsforschung in Cologne let me scan the treasures of their library, heeding my pleas.

 https://doi.org/10.11647/OBP.0331.14

Yet far away from my home shores I longed for familiarity, as so much made me restless and uneasy! The lack of meaningful work and teaching opportunities. The necessity to indiscriminately download the whole Taylor and Francis catalogue, because the INION[1] library in Moscow only provided paid access by the hour. The looming morass of bullshitting that I encountered during my university studies—although that was comfortable for quite a few across the board—from the humble abodes of the Russian State University for the Humanities (alma mater, I salute you!) to the palatial chambers of MGIMO.[2] The knowledge that a certain expert copies and pastes from Claudio Radaelli without citing him. The increasingly widespread ideological servitude at the behest of the powers that be. All these things made me shiver in dread!

It was not all doom and gloom, for I have glimpsed the truly skillful, the astute and the humane. Fondly I keep in my memory the advice of N, whom I owe a lot, the remarks of Y, the discussions with G, the lectures of P, the wisdom of S, as well as innumerable gifts of others. Yet too few were they to calm the churning waters, so I set sail!

I was awe-stricken upon arrival. The lands of the Belgae and the Batavians held untold riches. Savants, about whom you had only read, appear before your own eyes, scriptoriums and tabulariums full to the brim. The sweet taste of empirical research rushes like adrenalin through your blood as you track and chase a new unsuspecting interviewee. Your spirit soars; you embrace the opportunity structure, and wings unfold behind your back.

O, San Precario, you bear witness that from the humble labors I have not turned away! Scores of BAs and MAs I have instructed, the multi-headed Hydra of the Liberal Arts and Sciences I have tamed, the bridges between the quan and the qual I have built, as well as—with your grace—the miracle of 'turning Brussels sprouts into French fries' I have executed, making research methods courses 'edible' for the student multitude.

Have I not explored the broadways and side-streets of European Union Studies Avenue, International Relations Boulevard, Comparative Politics Lane, International Political Economy Drive? Have I not tested

---

1    A large social science library in Moscow that later partially burned down, potentially due to real estate interests.
2    Quite a posh and prestigious institution that—amongst other things—prepares Russian diplomats.

my mettle when competing for the hand of the beautiful lady Veni[3] and the incomparable lady Curie?[4] (I will soon find a lady much finer than you two!) Have I not committed the glorious folly of publishing beyond the topic of my PhD?

Too late I have seen that, even in the garden of earthly delights, Precarity lies in wait! I was haunted by the short-term contract. By the realization that the making of a course can be equated with chopping a book into chapters and sprinkling it with a couple of articles. By the prearranged job openings. By the fact that a small amount of money for fieldwork is more difficult to get than a large NWO[5] grant. By the advice to cut down the costs of a policy event to such an extent that the event makes sense no more.

The heart of mine trembled in fear, for the very Precarity I was running away from stood towering before me, blotting out the sun. For the very things that I thought were privy to the region I came from were (and are) in full blossom here! And it saddened my heart, and I was cast low. For too much do I love and respect my craft to cut corners. I would abandon it, rather than fake it.

So, with a heavy heart I cast my net wide, getting ready to sell myself to the Albert Heijn corporate store, to enlist into the call center for gamers and abandon academia for good.

Yet, in those days of sorrow you did not abandon me, o, San Precario. An odd job at Clingendael,[6] a report on a conference here, a pep-talk from colleagues and friends there have kept my spirits up and running. And then it dawned on me that I was not the only itinerant academic, for many, far too many, walked the same sorrowful road. Exhausted from combining several 0,3 fte contracts, given no credit for enthusiastic teaching, cast into a semi-eternal whirlpool of visiting lectureships, sacrificing personal life for the ephemeral benefit of yet another paper, 'hazed' for coming from far-away regions of the Orient (which is anywhere between Germany's eastern borders and Australia)—in such a state are my fellow academics.

'Is there a way out?', questioned I.

---

3    A type of Dutch national individual research grant.
4    Here I refer to the Marie Curie research grant.
5    NWO—Dutch Research Council, a national body responsible for research fund allocation.
6    Clingendael Netherlands Institute of International Relations.

To the streets I took, waving the red banner of WOinactie[7] and pinning their emblem to my back-pack. Proudly I bear it to this day. We—the participants of the demonstrations—have not demanded 'More Money!', for just throwing money at a problem rarely solves anything. We demanded more long-term and permanent contracts, alongside an end to the de-coupling of teaching and research (as if you could split yourself in half and carry on living), smaller and smarter funding schemes rather than only the gargantuan grants, for which everyone competes with a close-to-zero success rate. Surprisingly, few senior potentates took to the streets with us, and they remained largely silent. Not many have heeded the living conditions of the academic precariat!

However, how can you be creative if survival is the sole focus of your daily chores?! How can you toil with no respite and without degrading yourself to a beast of burden, voiceless and stupefied from hard labor? Yet it is free time, security, and peace of the heart that allows us to thrive and indulge in intellectual experiments. While precarity deprives us of our creativity.

Would Stefano Mancuso have been inspired about plant intelligence were he not allowed to watch Star Trek? For you may see Bertrand Russell as a cuckoo, but 'In Praise of Idleness' he does have a point! (And I should thank Student 1 for indirectly and unwittingly making me acquainted with this text.) Or could one actually read (not scroll through, but slowly and diligently read) all the recommended literature for a course of one's own design if consistently under the Damocles sword of a non-renewable contract? Wouldn't a student know more, wouldn't an instructor be able to engage with the mosaic of human knowledge and further extend and embellish our common heritage, if only a longer time period was given? Even game theory teaches us that players cooperate if the game is repeated, dedicating themselves and building trust if only they don't live by the day! Then why is all this neglected?

What am I, San Precario, within this maelstrom? What will become of me? What awaits my academic companions?

Truly, there is 'neither Jew nor Gentile', to quote a Bible verse, as our background and origin do not predetermine what is to become of us. Being of Russian origin is as much about loving vodka, bears,

---

7    An informal civic movement in the Netherlands that tries to fight against long-term cuts and deteriorating working conditions in the Dutch university education.

and Kalashnikov machine guns as being from India is about fancying Bollywood, curry, and joining the Holi festival. Too often our birthplace is a nametag, to say it mildly, or a stereotype, to say it bluntly, that others use to wrongly make sense of us. I have seen 'Westerners' engage in Byzantine politics of epic proportions, and I have witnessed 'Easterners' stick to the rules of integrity and transparency for no personal gain. Neither is it one's degree and place within the hierarchy: with my own eyes I have seen postgraduates perform such miracles of faith that would be beyond the reach of some associate professors! It must be something else then, fluid and intangible. 'Know we too well that this challenge has no solution yet esteem we to find conditions under which it is possible,' I quote the S brothers.

Consider, San Precario, a metaphor, for I am an admirer of such mind-games, like the Buddhist monks with their *koans*. Truly, it is within our power to produce all the food we need. Yet, famine persists, and malnutrition is rife. Hence, it is how we set up our supply chains, market stalls, and distribution criteria that affects the hunger. It can be done differently. So it is with academia, I think, o beloved San Precario! It can be done differently! Academia can be different! If in the face of eternity Jan Blommaert could say so, so can we—we who still wander this world.

Am I warped by my travels, without perspective, out of touch with my roots, as was claimed by some? No, San Precario, I am not, for I was like this long before I set sail. Less naïve am I, that is true, much more cynical, aware of the complexity of this world, bearing my hard-won scars with pride; yet I have not lost my core. Deeply I lament my parting with the country of my birth (and even more, my parents' home) back in 2010, yet I cannot condone the things that have been done in my home country over the past years and in foregone times. What do I feel, you will ask, when I come across a taxi driver or a tea seller from Afghanistan with a PhD in engineering from the USSR in 1970s? I am appalled, for I see first-hand a little glimpse of the events that unchained so much suffering for no reason at all. What of the war with Ukraine? What of the misery? What of the lost time?

Am I, San Precario, a descendant of a Vyatich or a Kryvich, am I a Batavian, am I a highly skilled migrant, an academic condotierre ready to fight for the highest bidder? I think I am all that and more. Above all, I am me. Under no flag but my own, fully aware that any flag is a social construction. And I console myself with a rumor that, were Rumi's parents not fleeing from yet another invasion into Afghanistan, there would be no Rumi. Move you must, even if it is hard.

What shall I pray for, San Precario? Will there be deliverance from precarity?

O, San Precario, even Shrek and Princess Fiona know that 'happily ever after' is not as straightforward as it may seem and is by no means 'the end of history.' Ultimately, it is not vengeance against individuals within the academic system that I desire—for violence will just breed more violence and things will remain the same. What I wish for is vindication. Not of my efforts, but of the efforts of the academic precariat across disciplinary boundaries! For far too many people were traumatized, far too much hardship and deprivation experienced, far too much injustice caused! Far too much unsubstantiated arrogance shown by those unaffected by the elements outside, those pent up in the ivory towers!

So, San Precario, join me in prayer, implore the ecumenical Almighty with me:

> Great is the Ocean and unfathomable are its riches,
> Beyond any measure it is, beyond control it is, limitless it is,
> Wise, sentient, and unforgiving it is,
> Majestic is its rolling beauty at any time of day and night,
> It brings joy to the heart and the eye, it warms the soul
> To cross it, courage and skill and understanding are much needed
> Without the Ocean you can neither be, nor do
> Yet harsh and merciless may life be, unforeseen is the fate
> It may cast you away from the Ocean to a waterless desert, or snowy mountains
> In fact, you may never see the Ocean again (or at all)
> Yet NEVER shall you act as if the Ocean does not exist
> You shall not act as if it's a folly of a madman
> You shall not pretend that it is not out there
> You shall not tell those under your guidance that it's a mere mirage
> Even though you may be laughed at and ridiculed
> Like a seashell that is cast from the waters, may you keep the Ocean within you
> And rejoice, when you find yourself on its shores once again'
> What do I wish for myself, San Precario?
> To fulfil something that Master NK wished a long time ago: 'Never stop!'

Amen!

# GENDERED PRECARITY AND SEXUALIZATION

.

# 15. Survival in Silence: Of Guilt and Grief at the Intersection of Precarity, Exile, and Womanhood in Neoliberal Academia

*Aslı Vatansever*

*Trigger warning: The chapter details an episode of sexual assault.*

The crisp July evening is filled with melancholic cheerfulness. Music in the background is slowly dying, overstatements of friendship and mutual affectio fly around. We are already lamenting the passing of this night; the present is already a memory, as our minds slowly depart towards impending return flights, upcoming summer vacations, next year's projects. To ward off the heavy air of farewell, overoptimistic plans are made to meet at this-and-that international conference here-or-there, whenever wherever. Little does anyone know at that point that, within less than a year, all those trips and conferences will turn into Zoom meetings. In less than a year, we will have understood that all those in-person meetings could have been emails, after all. But right now, we are all in that mood that only summer farewells can put you in: a state of sensitive vibrance, a sort of wistful optimism.

I'm on my third glass of wine and my third year in exile. I'm not tipsy but somewhat intoxicated by the blues of a whole year gone by. As is the rule in the hyper-mobile 21st-century academia, I am practically used to farewells exactly around this time of the year, every year. Except this time, I'm the one staying behind for a change. People I met this year are

https://doi.org/10.11647/OBP.0331.15

either going back to their home institutions or transferring to someplace else. I don't have an institution or a home to go back to. I'm staying put in my main exile station, Berlin. Somehow stationary yet eternally in transit. Formally safe but substantially precarious.

I am sad, but also kind of relieved for not having to move internationally, as I had done every summer for the last three years. This time, I'm only moving within the city, to another apartment. Finding an apartment in Berlin is a nightmare known to anyone who has ever lived here. Moving apartments, alone, without a car or a helping hand, will be my individual horror story that I allow myself not to think about tonight. By the beginning of summer, when it became clear that I was going to have to move from my sublet soon, on a dare, I had made a bold and contradictory decision to finally ship my entire household from Istanbul to Berlin, knowing that this time I would not sublet but rent a long-term apartment. It was a bold decision, because I didn't have a job except for a one-year extension of my current fellowship, and there was no possibility of any sort of life stability in sight. And it was a contradictory decision, too, because I hate the city with all my heart—I always did, even before exile—and it's the last place I'd want to settle and spend the rest of my life in, even if I had the chance to do so. But I had grown tired of living in guesthouses, sublets, with stuff that wasn't mine. I couldn't stand the thought of letting my entire life perish in a dark storage room anymore, waiting for me to go back and reclaim it, like an abandoned baby at the doorsteps of a mosque. I was done suspending time. I was tired of keeping my finger pressed on the 'pause button,' so I decided to not only resume but flash forward while I could.

On that July evening I know that I'm still hanging by a thread, but I'm desperately trying to make that thread a bit more appealing for myself. I'm lingering on—but lingering on a little more firmly every year. I work better the less I believe that hard work will bring anything at the end. The less I see a future, the more strongly I attend to the present. The less I wish to settle here, the more I get used to the soul-crushing dullness of this stationary. So, I stay put that summer and for the foreseeable future. I make plans to move my old life from Istanbul to Berlin. I am waiting for the results of my seven-hour-long asylum interview with the Migration Office a few months back. In dispassionate lucidity and proper German, I had explained for seven hours how and why the social contract between the Turkish state and me has been breached for good. The fact that I had to struggle to obtain the right to stay in a place I don't even want to stay in is the kind of cruel irony you would find in Gogol. But I never expected a Jane Austen type of jolly satire from my life, anyway.

Thus, at the onset of 'the summer of cruel ironies,' I find myself at this party. Inside, the hoopla is still in full swing. Outside on the terrace, I'm watching the belated sunset fade away behind the cityscape. People come out to smoke and then go back in to dance or get another drink. When I'm alone, I feel the famous summertime sadness like a papercut. Whenever people come by, I crack jokes and entertain everyone. Here, on the terrace, I find the perfect balance between extroverted socialization and introverted withdrawal. I hardly expect anything else from a social activity, anyway. Fun is not a prerequisite. Not since I went into exile, at least. And most certainly not in Berlin. In Berlin, any attempt to have actual fun beyond the predictable social pleasantries is more painful than the absence of fun itself. So, I'm sitting here serenely in my lack of genuine interest for anything or anyone. At one point, I find him sitting in a chair next to me. Suddenly, I feel his fingers moving on my thigh where I sit. A little farther over the other side of the terrace, there are people. *There are people around.* It's his indecent act but, somehow, I feel like I have something to hide. I move uncomfortably in my chair; I feel like I should cover this up on his behalf. *There are people around.* But the knowledge that men in power will always find a way to punish you for their own crimes is too deeply rooted. After all, everybody knows that he is a notorious sexual predator with past records of molesting female students, and the entire German academia has been willing to turn a blind eye to this for the sake of his shrewd sense for lucrative academic businesses.

Years and years of research on power relations and inequalities in academia, feminist teachings, my otherwise assertive flair and combative exterior—and all I manage to blurt out is a pathetic 'you know, this makes me uncomfortable.' I get up softly to avoid suspicion and go mingle with the other people. I feel guilty for some reason. Why did I act so vaguely? Am I scared of the consequences? Scared that a loud and scandalous rejection might cost me my affiliation which I need so badly for my residence permit, my asylum application, and my next round of funding? Could I be that small? Or could the will to survive in a hostile environment, no matter what, be so big? No, it can't be so dramatic. I surely must be overthinking for no reason. I keep telling myself that nothing significant happened. I keep telling myself that it's late and we're all a bit too loose. I relativize the surreal memory of his fingers on my thigh a minute ago. I whitewash his misdeed on his behalf, for my own peace of mind. After all, there are people around. If it were such a big deal, he wouldn't have dared to do such a thing in public, would he? *There are people around*. Their existence is my reality check.

I'm making the rounds, talking to those other people who are my sole anchor to solid reality at this point. He is following me wherever I go. Sometimes with his eyes, sometimes physically. I don't read too much into it. He is drunk and he is generally a vulgar and impudent type. People don't mind. The entire German academic community doesn't mind. I, an absolute nobody with no protective professional or personal ties around here, shouldn't mind either. Soon, I decide to take off and say goodbye to a few people. Loud and chaotic farewells, big hugs, promises to keep in touch and meet then-and-there, thanks and good wishes getting thrown around all over the place.

> Who will clean up this mess?—Ah, the poor cleaning lady, shall we at least throw away the bottles?—No, no.—You're leaving already?—Man, we drank a lot!—I'm gonna miss you so much!—You guys, we will definitely come to Berlin next summer.—I can't believe you don't have Facebook!—Are you going to keep your WhatsApp number when you get back?—I'll be around for another week.—Oh my God, we should totally meet before you leave!—Love youuuu!!
>
> Aslı, could you come to my office for a sec? I want to show you something.

When I get out of that office, I am not the same person who went in. There are still people around. There were people around, too, when I was in that office for probably four to five minutes, biting his tongue when he forcefully stuck it into my mouth, pushing him away, struggling to rid myself off his bearish grasp, biting the arm with which he was squeezing my breast. There were people around, they were supposed to be my reality check. But behind that closed door, he obviously possessed the power to suspend reality. Outside, there were people, when, inside, I was fighting, both physically and with strategic remarks on how inappropriate it was, or would be, if he pursues this. For some reason, I am trying to act as if all he did was to ask me out on a date. I remain ice-cold throughout the episode. Because somehow, I cannot bring myself to see myself in a victim role. I am habitually not afraid of uninvited sexual advances in social situations. I keep telling myself I can fend off anything, as long as I'm not kidnapped at gunpoint, thrown into a van, and raped in a dark corner, which, by the way, is a frighteningly possible scenario for all women, at any given time. What actually throws me off at this moment is my own cold-blooded reaction. There is something disgusting in the way I never lose sight of the register of power relations I'm entangled in. Something feels off in the way I maintain a sociopathic detachment during the hurly-burly. Impulsively yet shrewdly, I try to make it look like a negotiation—as if there is anything to negotiate. I try to act with a high sense of power—as if I still possess some sort of leverage and control over the situation. He literally uses brutal, physical force.

A surreal scenery, an absurdly non-epic battle, a close-up from Rubens' 'Rape of the Sabine women' reincarnated for the 21st-century German academia: a foreign female guest researcher in exile struggling to fight off a senior German professor in his office, biting and kicking around, trying to release herself from his violent grasp, but keeping her calm and full composure all the while, telling him placidly that her life is hard enough the way it is, in order to subliminally signal authority and tranquility, as if they're sitting and talking over a glass of wine. If the abduction of the Sabine women was a tragedy, this ambush he set up in his office is a bitter farce: the banality and grossness of an old man in power, forcing himself onto women in lower academic positions, unable to contain himself even with people in immediate proximity, confident that his title grants him the same rights as a feudal lord in late Middle Ages. And his confidence is not at all unsubstantiated: full professors in Germany indeed possess virtually the same rights over their precarious juniors as a feudal lord did over his serfs. The German academic system is a broken time-machine, where medieval hierarchies and feudal bonds co-exist alongside the 21st-century neoliberal mechanisms of labor devaluation. Just a few months after this incident, one of my interviewees for my project on precarious academic workers in Germany will use the exact same words, when she says that 'the assistants are the serfs of their professors.'

But right now, there are people outside. Just outside that door. You could hear them talking. Weird that I don't even think of them in that moment. I don't even think of alarming them; for some reason, making a scene in the middle of the academic community does not even exist as an option in my mind. So detached is the image of the academic business from the day-to-day abominations that occur in its shadowy hallways and locked offices. Just like we are convinced that the job insecurity we face in academia is something we need to overcome individually by working harder, publishing more, and beating our rivals, somewhere along the line, I must have subconsciously internalized the idea that I'm completely alone in this hostile environment and have to deal with workplace misconduct and sexual harassment from seniors on my own. A perfect combination: the 21$^{st}$-century individualization of misery meets the archaic patriarchal tradition of woman-blaming.

I get out of that office with a victory that doesn't feel like one. Yes, I did manage to ward off his assault. But I feel like the way I did so has corrupted a part of my soul. I feel like I'm complicit. I feel like I acted out of character. I feel like I'm decadent and cunning. I feel like I should have lost my calm in there and shaken the entire building with my screams for help. I feel like I shouldn't have tried to appear powerful. I should have let myself become the victim, so that he could be exposed as the villain he was. But I stayed calm, despite the wrestle, in a subconscious act of refusal to accept the power dynamic that a sexual assault imposes upon the victim. Even though I was subjected to physical assault and literally had to engage in a visceral fight, *I failed to feel vulnerable.* I failed to feel and act like a woman under assault. *I failed to feel and act like a woman.*

But maybe it wasn't exactly 'out of character'. After all, I had been accused of *unwomanly self-defense* in the past. Not awfully long ago, a senior male professor personally attacked me in a colloquium and publicly discredited my work for having a Marxist approach. Instead of bending in and sugarcoating my arguments in the usual accommodating submissiveness that is often expected from non-tenured female faculty, I had assertively and systematically refuted his subjective insults disguised as critique. Yet, while trying to fortify my arguments, the necessity to 'feminize' my mode of argumentation must have escaped me. Later on, I heard how one female colleague tried to defend me afterwards by drawing attention to the stark power asymmetry in that debate, whereas another female co-worker is said to have argued condescendingly that I don't *deserve* feminist solidarity, for I am obviously capable of defending myself 'like a man' against men. In any case, this had been a real eye-opener for me: in some people's eyes, to be worthy of feminist solidarity (or any solidarity, for that matter), you had to act the part, you had to let your wounds bleed and your voice tremble.

As a matter of fact, being an exiled 'scholar at risk,' I was familiar with such expectations. The rules of the game of professional solidarity have been all too clear in recent years. Haven't I been asked the same questions about 'what I've been through' over and over again, in every interview, at every conference, with the same appetite in the correspondents' eyes to rub the wounds they assumed were there? Wasn't the entire academic risk industry—which I, like many other fellow Peace Academics, had been greatly dependent on for the last few years—based on this type of victimization and pornography of pain? Occasions might vary, but solidarity, as long it is not the result of an organic collective struggle but offered as an act of generosity, is universally (and patronizingly) premised on the injured party's helplessness and conformity to victim stereotypes: you have to build your whole identity around your wound, or else your wound is not real. If you don't show where it hurts, no one will trust that it hurts. If you carry it too well, no one will believe how heavy your burden is. Patronage disguised as solidarity. Clientele disguised as collectivity.

I go out to the hallway. I'm relieved to see that there are still people around. As if I had been in there for hours. People in the hallway don't seem to suspect anything. But why do I care whether they find out or not? Why do I feel like I have to hide what happened? Why did I fight a secret battle inside and why am I still trying to cover it up? *There are people around.* If I had made a scene inside and screamed for help, they could have heard and come to my rescue. Why didn't I? Am I, in my reluctance to expose his act, justifying it? Did my passive reaction to his fingers on my thigh invite him to lock me in, force his alcohol-reeking tongue into my mouth, and grope me? At that moment, all I can think of is to go get my coat and my purse from my office as fast as I can and get the hell out of the building. While I'm running to my office at an unsuspicious speed, I quickly calculate in my mind various trivial things like a habitual sociopath: 'I had said goodbye to most people before he duped me into his office, so I don't have to make the rounds again—this saves me time so I can get out more quickly'; 'Shall I take the fire exit, in order to avoid the risk of bumping into him in the elevator? But the staircase is too deserted at this hour; it could be even more dangerous if he catches me there,' and so on.

I reach my floor; it's dark and empty. *There are no people around.* This means I have entered the zone of horrible surreal possibilities again. I am frightened and nervous, although, in my mind, I gravitate towards the comfort of self-doubt. I am already downplaying what happened. I am discrediting my own recollection of what just happened, telling myself I am being too dramatic. He did not rape me. I did not scream. I did not cry. I even doubt that I responded harshly enough. So, it must be nothing. But then again, why am I terrified to be alone in an empty floor right now? My heart is pounding as I make the fastest ever packing-up round in my office. Again: *Staircase or elevator? Staircase or elevator? Think but think fast.* There are people downstairs. They might take the elevator, too. Elevator is safe. Safer than the fire exit. Elevator is fast and good. Elevator it is then.

The fact is, at that point, two choices unfold in front of me, each more degrading than the other. The first option is to adopt a gendered and victimized mode of defense, which, for some reason, has always seemed like something ill-proportioned and unjustified for me. Something that I don't deserve with my impenetrable exterior and seeming invulnerability. I can never deem myself aggrieved enough to justify a call for help. I don't deserve compassion unless I'm shaken to my core. I am not worthy of feminist solidarity unless I'm completely crushed. I don't qualify as a woman in my feminist comrades' eyes, as long as I am capable of beating men in their own game. The second option is to own up to my allegedly watertight imperviousness to male toxicity, to tone down my anger and pain, and to convince myself that I am complicit in what happened to me, because I didn't let it destroy me. I am not as broken as a victim should be after a sexual assault. By virtue of resilience, I am the enabler of my own abuse. An intolerantly self-responsible form of agency, a punitive self-centeredness, a self-condemning mode of subjectivation: that's my comfort zone.

Thus, with the past insight on feminist solidarity criteria engraved in my mind, knowing that my demeanor categorically disqualifies me as injured party, I start to gaslight myself. In the days and months following that night, I feel obliged to keep things gracious. I reply to his emails in a lighthearted—even sympathetic—way as if what happened that night was a flirtatious joke. I endure his presence on multiple occasions, once even at my own place along with other guests, only a few days after that incident, because I couldn't take the risk of causing a diplomatic scandal by disinviting him. But in the background, I cling to a young, precarious female colleague like myself the entire evening—in my own house!—telling her what happened the other day and begging her to stay with me until everybody (i.e., he) leaves. She does. She stays long after everybody leaves, letting me relax and shake off the anxiety of that night, talking about this and that, not once asking why I didn't scream and call for help in that office, not even slightly implying that I might have 'asked for it,' not denying me feminist solidarity for not acting 'wounded' enough.

To this day, I keep that corrupt friendly façade. I remain decadently outgoing. The more I do this, the more I loathe and blame myself for not being more unambiguous. And the more I keep this nonchalance, the less I see myself as justified to take a clean cut as time passes by. As if the real crime is not sexual harassment on the assailant's part per se, but paralysis on the attacked person's part. As if men are not to blame for unsolicited sexual advances, but women are to blame when they fail to scream loud enough. Even in cases where there is a clear power asymmetry and no trace of consent in any way, if a man makes a move and you fail to let him harm you enough to make a public scandal out of it immediately, you will forever be subjected to the violence of public suspicion. So, instead of delivering my head to that guillotine of backhanded victim-blaming, I retreated to a cunning-calculative mode of self-defense and executed myself, with my own hands, a million times in my mind since then.

In retrospect, I often thought: 'He wouldn't have dared to do this if I were a full professor!' As true as this assumption is, focusing on the academic power dynamic must have appeared more soothing to me in its ordinariness, than thinking about the disturbing question *'what could have, would have, happened, if there weren't any people around* in the hallway?'. But maybe the solution to our individualized grievances lies herein anyway: in asking what happens every day, in countless offices and hallways, in a hierarchical industry and exploitative work culture like this. And how the contingent faculty majority—those who do not know someone who knows someone who knows someone, those who do not have an elite alma mater or an influential benefactor, those who were born in one of the 'wrong' countries and do not possess the 'right' passport, women, migrants, people with a lower-middle class background, LGBTQI, people with disabilities or politically marginalized approaches—must be enduring all sorts of workplace misconduct by their seniors. And how many of them must be blaming themselves, feeling that a part of them has been irreversibly corroded and degenerated by a survival in silence.

# 16. To the Center and Back: My Journey Through the Odds of Gendered Precarity in Academia

*Emanuela Mangiarotti*

My essay reflects on how my experience of reintegrating into Italian academia was chiefly defined by my identity as a homecoming female researcher, and how moving back from a ten-year-long stay abroad made me radically aware of how gender marks the endemic precarity of cultural work within the European university system. I use an autobiographical lens, which runs through some of the moments and contexts of my life in the university, centering on my experience of moving from the center space of British academia to the relative margins of the Italian one.

My narrative revolves around the issue of mobility: my experience of entering certain academic spaces as a female 'native' returnee whose academic trajectory had crossed disciplinary boundaries. While centered on my own specific circumstances and lived experience, and without a claim to speak for others, I situate my own personal journey within the paradigm of gendered precarity[1] and draw inspiration from existing literature about the contextual, contingent, and differential forms of vulnerability of transnational professional trajectories in neoliberal academia. I thus aspire to make a contribution to the growing conversation taking place among women cultural workers, which was initiated by intersectional, queer, and decolonial feminists, about

---

[1] On gendered precarity in the academic system see Zheng (2018); Morley (2018); Murgia and Poggio (2019). For a focus on the Italian context see Bozzon, Murgia, Poggio, and Rapetti (2017); Poggio (2017).

 https://doi.org/10.11647/OBP.0331.16

our peculiar positionality in the relations of super/subordination that pervade and sustain academic spaces.

## Out of place

*I land in Belgium, at the Brussels-based campus of a UK university's IR department, thinking: 'What if they made a mistake?' I learn to live with the impostor syndrome throughout much of my PhD experience, especially in contexts where (I thought) I should come across as smart and 'at ease'... in English. That is the case also in social gatherings with colleagues and senior scholars which—I begin to understand—make up an important part of building my academic persona. 'Manu, you're too anxious! You should try yoga!' suggests a male, native Anglophone colleague of mine. I do try yoga in the end, although not thanks to his advice but because, together with some of my PhD girlfriends, I decide that yoga could be a good way to address our common doctorate-related stress and have something that brings us together outside university. It does indeed help, as our friendship grows, and we build solidarity and a sense of community as young and 'anxious' migrant women trying to navigate precarious but exciting early careers in the knowledge production industry in the heart of Europe.*

I have come to understand this specific kind of anxiety as a sense of being 'out of place.' Rachele Borghi describes the 'out of place syndrome' as the internalization of the perspectives of dominant voices and the concurrent feeling of occupying a material or symbolic public space illegitimately (Borghi, 2020, 47). In my experience, trying to feel 'in place' when you struggle to adapt to new worldviews, scientific paradigms, languages, and scholarly habitus can be tiring and disorienting (ibid. 47–48). Indeed, as a Southern European (white) woman, adapting to the dominant academic center-space (a UK postgraduate school of international studies) often unsettled my sense of self and, at times, made me question my legitimacy as an aspiring researcher. Part of it was linked to my poor understanding of the taken-for-granted language, habits, and tastes that make up recognizable academic lifestyles and that, indeed, can be regarded as forms of cultural capital.[2] The topic of my PhD research did not help either. In an IR department, I pursued

---

2    On the dominance of English and anglophone universities in academic knowledge production, see Curry and Lillis (2007); Marton (2019); Nota (2020).

an ethnographic study of communal conflicts in India, with a gender focus and a feminist epistemology. A male English senior scholar I had previously and very briefly worked with once said: 'You actually managed to pull off that project?!' He seemed awkwardly surprised.

## Getting there

*I actually pass my PhD viva without corrections—a rather rare occurrence in British academia. I feel rewarded and—for some time—relieved of the out-of-place syndrome. I have actually made it. 'She defended her dissertation in a remarkably undefensive way' I find written on the examiners' report. This remark brings me back to the feeling of calm and confidence I felt as I sat in front of them, rooted in the awareness of my path and the choices I had made to make the project work both for me (a feminist scholar) and for them (who had to judge it based on the assessment standards peculiar to the UK academic system). I especially remember how feminism had opened me up to the possibility that feeling out of place could turn into a sense of hanging in the right place, finding the political in the personal and seeking to connect with those who, in the end, questioned—and fought against—the normality of privilege.*

Feminist bonds have shown me that feeling out-of-place is tiring but can feed into our political consciousness. It can lead us to ask questions about why what is normal does not feel right. It might eventually make us feel that, when we start questioning how things are, we will continue to struggle but will find ourselves in very good company. According to Borghi (2020, 14), this process of understanding your positioning as a political issue has to do with unmasking the tacit ways in which academic authority and power are differentially distributed based on interlocking systems of oppression. Gender and class, of course, matter, but they cannot be separated from whiteness and country of origin in a knowledge production industry that channels internationalization in specific directions that usually uphold center-periphery dynamics (Marton, 2019). So, from there, the lens through which I looked at my personal struggles became inevitably political. I began to recognize the privilege of my Belgian residence permit, as a white, middle-class European 'pondering her options' after completing the PhD, but I also started to realize the specific way in which gendered precarity was becoming a defining aspect of my post-PhD life as a female, unemployed migrant academic.

# Coming home

*After a ten-year-long stay in Belgium, my partner and I decide to go back to Italy (our native country) with our two-year-old baby girl. I am somewhat ambivalent about moving. We love Brussels and we are surrounded by wonderful friends, but relationships feel potentially impermanent as our circles consist mostly of migrant professionals like us. At the same time, I feel excited at the idea of coming home, hoping I will find a job, capitalizing on my research and work experiences abroad. I break the news to colleagues and friends at the university. Encouragement, support, bittersweet goodbyes, and promises to stay in touch, and... 'Are you sure? I mean, you could end up like those educated, middle-class Italian women with a professional future in front of them until they have a baby, quit their jobs and start knitting and baking cakes while waiting for their husband at home!' I think my face shows my disbelief and uneasiness at this comment (rage mounts afterwards as I narrate the conversation to a friend of mine) because he quickly adds: 'Joking, of course!'*

Feeling diminished based on the interlocking dimensions of your social identity reveals how out-of-place syndrome is, indeed, a political issue. It is related to how privilege tacitly marks a person's sense of entitlement (or lack thereof) based on her positioning with respect to the norms that underscore relations of domination in the academic space (Borghi, 2020, 23, 44). I learned that the precarious feeling of fitting in, mediated by the possibilities which my social positioning as a white European opened for building up my cultural capital within UK academia, could be easily jeopardized, as the prospect of 'going back' activated commonly held gender and cultural stereotypes. When I recall my journey through academia, I describe out-of-place syndrome as a corporeal dimension of gendered precarity, which creeps into your core and manifests as uneasiness in interactions with senior colleagues and staff or even when entering university buildings, where your social identity somehow determines to what extent you belong, and whether or how you will have to prove you actually do.

# Options

*Employment prospects back home are dim, and the whole process of looking for options is tiring. I get a new PhD scholarship so that I can get paid for my research and realize—once again—that I am not alone. There are actually a few of us in the Italian university system: early-career scholars with a PhD obtained abroad, who come home and embark on a new PhD programme, in a different—although often akin—disciplinary field. And among them, the majority are women. I see a pattern taking shape: after short-term post-doc fellowships, publications, low-paid teaching contracts, exhausted by the prospect of endless precarity, many drop out, and some of them become schoolteachers. Many find motherhood very hard to reconcile with early-career academic life. I feel scared but determined to work myself through the precarity of Italian academia while I get to know the women—whom I will come to consider my 'sisters'—of the Italian feminist movement Non Una di Meno ('Not One Less'). By sticking with them and taking an active part in the movement, I become acutely aware that my struggle is personal in the way it translates into 'my life,' but exquisitely political in the way its dimensions match the struggles of many other women.*

*And I do register in the national schoolteachers' ranking lists; one never knows!*

It is hard not to think that perhaps the racist and sexist 'joke' that my colleague in Brussels made about Italian women with promising but aborted careers might actually be rooted in the fact that dropping out of academia because of gendered precarity has become normalized—it is just 'the way things are.' And the explanation I find, based on the feminist lens I wear, is that when a similar phenomenon gets 'taken for granted,' it has to do with the workings of a politico-economic regime where the division of labor is clearly gendered, racialized, and classed. Early-career female scholars are constantly reminded of their subaltern position through the material implications in terms of overwork, low pay, and exhaustion experienced when stepping into a male-dominated, androcentric space of knowledge production (Bagilhole and Goode, 2001). In that sense, life for female academic migrant returnees is not necessarily more difficult than for other female scholars in this academic space. However, the process of making your scholarly trajectory fit into the national academic system can add a layer of uncertainty, in terms of lacking the necessary contacts and understanding of the system, besides having to embark in time-consuming and expensive bureaucratic procedures for skill and qualification recognition.

## Engrained in the system

*I get a teaching contract as adjunct faculty. Many of us, early-career academic returnees, do it in order to set foot in the institutional setting. A senior fellow academic tells me that 'precarity is also an opportunity to make unconventional career choices,' but I am not sure how my current professional situation can be read as an opportunity to choose, as I do not see many available paths ahead of me. Patronizing comments, even if well-intended, are part of the things that make me feel out of place. I feel I should do something so that my international experience and my interdisciplinary background pay off. Yet, the worried expression of most of my colleagues when I tell them about my unusual academic trajectory—spanning from Area Studies to Feminist Theory and Sociology— rings an alarm bell: 'traveling across disciplinary boundaries is risky.' And it is indeed, in a scholarly environment that, despite the grand narrative about multi- and inter-disciplinarity, frames career progressions and appointments within separate and non-communicating fields. I now feel, ironically, deeply engrained in the normality of this neoliberal institutional setting: here I am, carrying out fundamental teaching almost for free, trying to build the necessary credentials to advance in my career, which (however) is fundamentally split between non- communicating disciplinary fields. I ask myself whether, by accepting to play into the system, I somehow contribute to reproducing this logic.*

The gendered logic of academic precarity plays a part when looking at the career conundrums of early-career researchers with paths that hardly conform to country-specific academic cultures. While 'internationalisation is a dominant policy discourse in higher education' as a 'major form of professional and identity capital in the academic labour market' (Morely et al., 2018, 538), transnational mobility is mired with uncertainty and insecurity in terms of life trajectories. Moreover, flexibility can certainly open doors to short-term appointments in multiple academic settings, but can sometimes turn into an obstacle to career progress, contributing to engraining precarity in academic employment practices. According to Robin Zheng, the main issues confronting contingent faculty come from their condition of 'cheap, flexible and disposable' workforce (2018, 236). For women in particular, this kind of precarity in academia often means juggling different, low- paid tasks while managing home life. While Zheng looks specifically at the US system, her observations resonate with the situation of many Western academic contexts (Murgia and Poggio, 2019). In the end, continues Zheng, some painstakingly make it, but many keep floating just above the surface for a very long time and—sometimes—decide it is simply not worth it.

## Finding your tribe

I look at my journey to the center space and back to the relative periphery of academia as a path towards understanding how each personal story is situated in a complex nexus of relations that, in the end, reveal the workings of privilege in the gendered, racialized, and classed European university system. My approach is now quite pragmatic: I see the way I am privileged enough to still be able to choose whether to stay or to leave academia, and the way my personal struggles are informed by my identity as a female migrant academic. The best piece of advice I have received so far came from Cassandra Ellerbe, a Black feminist scholar and social activist based in the Netherlands, who once said to me in an informal conversation: 'the only way to survive and, perhaps, to finally thrive, is to find your tribe.' It's proven to be true. Although I keep struggling with time issues, torn between publication deadlines, teaching, conference presentations, and childcare, I have made time for feminist connections within and without the university. I have discovered vibrant, diverse, and committed communities of feminist scholars who dare to break the rules: they get together, organize, exchange information, work together, transform scientific paradigms, and support each other in the process of navigating the realm of academic (gendered) precarity. Taking care of oneself and others goes against some of the disconcertingly demeaning and taken-for-granted mantras of academic success and competition (e.g., 'publish or perish'). I cherish the feeling of mutual recognition that I experienced after reading the thoughtful comments and suggestions from a friend and feminist researcher on a chapter she volunteered to read. I have learnt it is possible to carve out safe spaces for critique but that it is even better when they turn into possibilities for alternative—although still marginal—academic practices. I have realized that the material implications of gendered precarity still bear on the extent to which I will be able to hang in there, but that, in the meantime, it is possible to live through it by building niches of resistance.

# Works cited

Barbara Bagilhole and Jackie Goode, 'The contradiction of the myth of individual merit, and the reality of a patriarchal support system in academic careers,' *European Journal of Women's Studies* 8/2 (2001): 161–180. https://doi.org/10.1177/135050680100800203

Rachele Borghi, *Decolonialità e privilegio: Pratiche femministe e critica al sistema-mondo* (Meltemi, 2020).

Rossella Bozzon, Annalisa Murgia, Barbara Poggio, and Elisa Rapetti, 'Work-life interferences in the early stages of academic careers: The case of precarious researchers in Italy', *European Educational Research Journal* 16/2–3 (2017): 332–351. https://doi.org/10.1177/1474904116669364

Mary Jane Curry and Theresa Lillis, 'The dominance of English in global scholarly publishing', *International Higher Education* 46 (2007), 6–7. https://doi.org/10.6017/ihe.2007.46.7948

Démeter Marton, 'The world-systemic dynamics of knowledge production: The distribution of transnational academic capital in the social sciences,' *Journal of World-Systems Research* 25/1(2019): 111–144. https://doi.org/10.5195/jwsr.2019.887

Louise Morley, 'Gender in the neo-liberal research economy', in *Gender Studies and the New Academic Governance: Global Challenges, Glocal Dynamics and Local Impacts*, ed. by H. Kahlert (Springer, 2018), pp. 15–40.

Louise Morley, Nafsika Alexiadou, Stela Garaz, José González-Monteagudo, and Marius Taba, 'Internationalisation and migrant academics: The hidden narratives of mobility', *Higher Education* 76 (2018): 537–554. https://doi.org/10.1007/s10734-017-0224-z

Annalisa Murgia and Barbara Poggio, *Gender and Precarious Research Careers. A Comparative Analysis* (Routledge, 2019).

Orion Noda, 'Epistemic hegemony: The Western straitjacket and post-colonial scars in academic publishing', *Revista Brasileira de Política Internacional* 63/1 (2020), e007. https://doi.org/10.1590/0034-7329202000107

Barbara Poggio, 'Women and men in scientific careers: New scenarios, old asymmetries', *Polis, Ricerche e Studi su Società e Politica in Italia*, 1 (2017): 5–16. https://doi.org/10.1424/86077

Robin Zheng, 'Precarity is a feminist issue: Gender and contingent labor in the academy', *Hypatia* 33/2 (2018): 235–255. https://doi.org/10.1111/hypa.12401

# 17. A *Smart* Hot Russian Girl From Odessa: When Gender Meets Ethnicity in Academia

## *Olga Burlyuk*

To a mildly informed western European, a comfortable image of a woman from our region is the proverbial 'nanny—house maid—mandarins gatherer'. Or a chick with lips, eyelashes and hair (all fake) who came to Europe 'for work'. And when you are an IT specialist, a diplomat, a writer, a scholar, a lawyer—to many, you know, this is outright offensive… For it doesn't fit the available stereotype. [auth. translation]

Irena Karpa, *How to Marry as Many Times as You Want* (2020), p. 81

Experiences like this: they seem to accumulate over time, gathering like things in a bag, but the bag is your body, so that you feel like you are carrying more and more weight… I remember each of these occasions… as a sensory event that was too overwhelming to process at the time.

Sara Ahmed, *Living a Feminist Life* (2017), p. 23

My future husband and I met at a student conference in the days before smartphones, when Skype was a novelty and it cost a fortune to call a fixed number. So we wrote letters, lots of letters. Well, emails. And before long, my Dutch husband (then boyfriend) started getting endless internet commercials for 'hot Russian girls from Odessa' and 'best escort girls in Kiev'—as every other male foreigner spotted in any type of online interaction with the country. Offensive and annoying as these are (including the sheer formulation: if you must, at least have the decency to advertise U-k-r-a-i-n-i-a-n girls from ode-S-a and k-Y-I-v), the idea of Ukrainian women as a highly sexualized local product perseveres,

   https://doi.org/10.11647/OBP.0331.17

and is regularly fanned at the highest political levels. In 2009, US Vice-President Joe Biden remarked to President of Ukraine Viktor Yushchenko that there were 'so many beautiful women here [in Ukraine].' In 2011, President of Ukraine Viktor Yanukovych famously invited participants of the World Economic Forum in Davos to visit Ukraine in spring 'when it starts to get hot in the cities of Ukraine and the women begin to undress.' And in 2019, President of Ukraine Volodymyr Zelenskyy proudly spoke during his European tour of Ukrainian women as a good tourism 'brand' for the country.

But what becomes of this when a Ukrainian woman leaves Ukraine to orbit the academic circles? In this essay, I walk down memory lane and recollect my professional interactions at the intersection of gender and ethnicity, spanning 15 years (2006–2020) and offering a sketch of everyday sexism and gendered racism in academia.

# April 2006

I am participating in a student conference on public international law at the Moscow State Law Academy. We are given hard copies of the latest book by one of the Academy's professors. I don't remember how it got to that—perhaps, it was a joke?—but Sergei, a student from Saint Petersburg, inscribes the book for me. He writes, 'To a lovely Ukrainian girl' (*zamechatelnoy khokhlushke*), using the Russian pejorative word for a female Ukrainian. Reduced to a lovely-Ukrainian-girl-in-the-pejorative, I am suddenly not the delegate with one of the best presentations at the conference (it is the very end, so we can tell) or the person who performed better in the Ukrainian national championship of the Jessup International Law Moot Court Competition than he did in the Russian one (we compared our 'credentials' first thing, of course). I am extremely annoyed, but also significantly outnumbered (by men and by Russians), so I let it slide.

I donate this book to the library of my alma mater one day.

# July 2006

I am at The European International Model United Nations (TEIMUN) conference in the Hague, my very first trip to 'the West.' The plenary welcome meeting has just ended, and I find myself in a large crowd, being squeezed slowly through a narrow door opening. It's extremely hot, and I say just that: 'I am so hot, it's crazy!' Several male students around me (seemingly Dutch, but I can't tell) start laughing and mocking, 'Are you, now?!' Blissfully ignorant of the double-meaning of the word at the time, I have no idea what they are alluding to and don't see what's so funny about me feeling overheated.

It is much later that I learn all the sexual undertones of the words in English (countless, really) and carefully, self-consciously select and ration my words.

## August 2006

As the public international law junkie that I've become, I am on my way to Salzburg for the Salzburg Law School on International Criminal Law. The summer school is pretty expensive, so I travel by bus to reduce costs. As I board the bus Kyiv-Munich, my parents ask cautiously whether I am *absolutely* sure this school *actually* exists and is not part of an elaborate human trafficking scheme. I brush off the remark as ridiculous: I am 19 and know it all; and besides, I am the most internet-literate in the family and have done my due diligence.

At the Polish-Ukrainian border, however, as I enter the ladies' restroom covered wall-to-wall in *La Strada International* posters listing 'Signs your trip is a human trafficking scam,' I catch myself going carefully through the proposed checklist. I am further reassured in knowing that my cousin will pick me up in Germany and drop me off in Salzburg: an extra pair of eyes 'on location.' I hold my passport close to heart (literally) for the remainder of the bus ride.

## May 2007

Luckier with the Hungarians than with the Croatians the year before, our team gets visas to participate in the Central and Eastern European Law Moot Competition, hosted in Budapest this time. Given our past experience—and seeing as our team consists of five young female students who are neither married, nor employed, nor have substantial savings in the bank, nor own real estate (read: major migration risk category)—we are tense throughout the application process and exhale only as we collect our passports with visas glued in them.

And so we are on our way to Budapest. Having arrived at the Ukrainian-Hungarian border by train, we swap to a Hungarian mini-van for the final leg of the trip. The composition of our group—one 30-something-year-old male coach and five 20-year-old female students—makes us wonder, semi-jokingly and semi-concernedly, whether border patrols will take us for a pimp and his girls, 'travelling on business.' Tell a cat it's a dog a sufficient number of times, and it will start questioning itself.

On this occasion, we are spared the interrogation.

# April 2008

As a MATRA/MTEC scholarship holder, I am at a designated training session on communication in an international context, alongside other scholarship students from Central and Eastern Europe (I wonder whether the Dutch-German majority of students in our MA program have received training like this earlier, or are simply not considered to need it). We have a captivating session by a business coach, who, it turns out, is a Dutch man married to a Belarusian woman. The fact comes up during a coffee break, and one of the girls asks him in what way Eastern European women differ from Western European, in his opinion. He pauses for a moment and replies, 'In the elegant combination of professionalism and femininity. It is not one or the other: it can be both.' The girls nod approvingly, flattered. I have a flashback to the poster for the International Women's Day, reading 'Zeg NEE tegen schoonheid!' (Say NO to beauty!), which I saw earlier in the streets of Maastricht. I was perplexed in that moment as to what a woman's beauty or lack thereof had got to do with women's rights (I know better today...).

# July 2009

I am granted a three-year full doctoral scholarship by the University of Kent, Brussels campus, starting in September. The scholarship is very generous: it covers your tuition fees (already set at sky-high rates by UK universities back then) and a monthly allowance. Hooray! Only... you need to teach under the conditions of the scholarship (which eats away precious time from the short three years you've got), and the allowance is so low that you can barely live off it (in fact, it is set at the legally required minimum for being allowed residence in Belgium; yes, I checked).

If I were to live alone or if I had a family to support, I would have to decline. Luckily, my soon-to-be husband is there to support me financially, and I am willing to accept his support without feeling too bad about it, seeing as I am giving up my 'mergers and acquisitions career' in Ukraine (and the solid income that comes with it) for love. We joke that I am an Eastern European gold-digger *ad absurdum*: while I did marry a Westerner and end up as his dependent (partially, temporarily, and by mutual agreement, but still), ironically, I've been making much more money back home and, unlike my husband, have no outstanding student debt.

## 2010

'Do you miss home?'—'Of course I do! Thanks for asking.' [I am so grateful for this expression of empathy and solidarity...]

## September 2010

From the second year of my PhD onwards, I continuously do fieldwork in Brussels; it is rather convenient to be based in the field. Besides attending numerous policy events, I interview officials, politicians, policy experts, and occasionally other scholars—and I systematically try to 'intercept' those individuals who are based elsewhere and come to Brussels on business. Often, they (who are, in the vast majority, men) suggest we meet in the lobby of their hotel: a highly practical and rather innocent logistical solution. Except, it puts me (now 24) in an awkward position of the proverbial 'Eastern European woman waiting for someone in a hotel lobby.' I hate it. It's an ordeal to be eye-scanned by hotel staff and residents passing by. I can read the dilemma off their faces: 'She looks Slavic, but she is dressed formally and holds a notepad. What's that now?'

After several instances like this, I schedule these interviews at coffee places nearby, accepting background noise as collateral damage.

# 2011

'Are all Ukrainian women as beautiful as you?'—'Eh...' [smile awkwardly]

# February 2011

I am heading for fieldwork in Ukraine and, in preparation for expert interviews, I buy myself high-heeled elegant winter boots (yes, those exist) and a laptop-size patent leather handbag (I cannot afford real leather on my PhD scholarship); I have a coat and formal dresses already. I also get a haircut and devote an evening to a proper manicure (nail polish and all). I do this because I know that if I am to 'look decent' and 'be taken seriously' in professional circles in Kyiv—and not be too noticeable—flat shoes, a backpack, and a ponytail (my 'European look') won't do. It's bad enough that I am a young female.

All this gearing-up undeniably helps, but it does not preclude me from being addressed with an 'Olichka,' which is a diminutive for 'Olga' and is utterly inappropriate at my age and in a professional context, or from men acting excessively gallantly and kissing my hand when I'd only extended it for shaking, etc. The quickly forgotten (general tolerance for) open sexism in Ukraine repeatedly startles me, although I suspect I should feel 'treated like a woman for once' and grow a pair of wings... On this occasion, I choose to conform and pretend to ignore the whole thing: conducting interviews is my main objective, and my trip is but a few weeks anyway. To get on, I get along.

# 2012

'Do you miss home?'—'Of course I do!' [And now I am sad and homesick and off my game; thank you very much...]

# August 2012

My three-year PhD scholarship is about to end, but my dissertation is not ready for submission, so I decide to take the fourth, 'extension' year. I have the luxury to consider this option: I am married to an EU citizen who, moreover, is willing and able to support me financially—which gives me a legal right to reside in Belgium (rather than having to pack up and leave the day my scholarship ends), as well as the precious time to focus on completing my PhD (rather than looking frantically for a job, any job, to justify residence and make ends meet).

It will take a year to finish my PhD and almost another year to score a full-time paid post-doc position. Fast-forward eight years, and I find myself facing a similar situation yet again, as my second post-doc is running out.

# September 2012

I am at the annual UACES conference in Passau. I am on the panel, presenting the latest of my doctoral research; I am in the write-up year, so this is my opportunity to run findings by the community. In the hour and a half that it lasts, and especially during my own talk, I look around the room for eye contact with the audience and exchange occasional glances with the few familiar faces and those people—men and women—who seem particularly attentive to the discussion. My talk goes great. I feel 'young and fabulous.'

As the panel ends and I leave the room; a man from the audience who I haven't met before approaches me to ask if I'd like to grab a drink. Still very much absorbed by the panel, I take that for a wish to continue the discussion and reply that I am actually going straight to welcome drinks now, so we can talk there. 'No, I mean grab a drink just the two of us, later tonight,' he says. Oh, that kind of a drink. 'No, sorry, I wouldn't be up for that. But we can still chat at welcome drinks,' I reply in a tone as friendly as I can: there is no need to attack a guy simply for finding you interesting (my mom has taught me to reject suitors respectfully); and besides, since I don't know who he is, I don't know how bad of an enemy I'd be making. 'Oh. You looked me in the eyes during the panel, so I took that as an invitation.' Say what now?... 'Well, that was just me keeping eye contact with the audience, nothing beyond that, really.' To which he says, 'Oh no. You *did* look me in the eyes.' What I reply in my mind is this: 'Hey, back off! I am not interested. See a wedding ring on my finger, right here?! N-o-t-a-v-a-i-l-a-b-l-e. And anyways, you are what, 15–20 years older than me?!' (Better yet: married and with a baby, as will appear later!). What I reply with my mouth is this: 'Well, you must have misunderstood. I am going to welcome drinks now. See you around.'

'See you around'—that's its own problem. It is day one of a four-day conference, and our professional community is tiny, so I am sure to see him around at this conference and future ones too. After he approaches me again during the conference dinner the next evening (which is on a boat, of all places!) and inquires if I have a nice hotel room, I decide to play the part of an insecure PhD student and cling on to Tom, my supervisor, for the remainder of the conference, just to be safe. Luckily, Tom and I are on such good terms that I can tell him openly what the deal is.

Days and weeks after, I revisit the episode and scrutinize my behavior: did I look him in the eyes beyond the respectable? Did I do that to other people? How long is respectable for a woman, by the way? For an attractive woman? For an attractive Eastern European woman? Are these all set at different times: three seconds for a man, two for a woman, one for an attractive woman, zero for an attractive Eastern European woman? How do I keep eye contact in the future, or do I do without? Was I being too friendly? Am I that naïve? One lesson is clear: I need to keep bigger distance from people, especially from men.

Unexpectedly, keeping distance and avoiding eye contact at the time of writing is as easy as ever: one Zoom-Webex-Teams-you-name-it online meeting + two screens = look away from the camera the entire time.

[Fun fact: I note down this episode as the very first when I start writing this essay, and I write it up as the very last.]

## 2013

'Where are you from?'—'Ukraine.'—'Oh yeah, now I see it!'—'Eh...' [awkwardly]

## June 2013

I have successfully defended my PhD and started the active search for an academic job. While I am trying my luck with any and all Belgian universities (a madman's undertaking, given I did my PhD at a non-Belgian university), people are generously forwarding me academic vacancies in random countries, encouraging me to apply—and evidently assuming I should-could-would be willing to move anywhere, really, nomad and outsider that I am. I know they do this with good intentions and a realistic understanding of the academic job market. But I can't help but feel a mounting frustration at everyone's expectation that I move again and with ease, leaving behind the life that I'd built for myself in the past four years, dragging along my husband (or leaving him behind too?) and unavoidably delaying any plans the two of us might have for starting a family. At this point, I am firmly set at 'exhausting domestic remedies' first and deciding later whether I would rather leave Belgium or leave academia.

## 2014

'Do you miss home?'—'Of course I do!' [Wait, are you subtly suggesting my home country might not be worthy of being missed?..]

## July 2014

I collect my PhD diploma at the graduation ceremony in the magnificent Canterbury Cathedral, marking the beginning of my history (*her*-story, really) of not being addressed with my proper title, 'Doctor,' in a professional context: not by fellow academics, not by students. One day, eager to use the title at least somehow, I tick 'Dr' when booking a flight; it's a German airline, and they honor hierarchies and titles that signify them. My husband warns me it is medical doctors they are after and 'you really don't want to be called upon when someone gets a heart attack during the flight,' so I diligently switch to 'Ms' instead.

Years later, when a dear friend of mine gets her assistant professor appointment, I hurry to send her a postcard addressed to 'Prof. Dr. Name Surname,' hoping this will be the first piece of mail she gets in the new status.

A year later, when I get mine, she returns the favor.

## December 2014

I inform Jan, my supervisor, of my pregnancy. I am excited to share the good news and a little anxious about his reaction: I've only worked here for half a year, you see. He is genuinely happy for me and does not so much as hint at this being inappropriate. I am relieved. He promises all the support there can be and says he will contact the HR department to inquire straightaway: it appears I am the first academic staff member in the department to get pregnant in the 'unforgotten past,' so there is no institutional memory on what maternity leave regulations actually are. Not that there have been no female staff of childbearing age in the department; it's just that no one has gone for it, for reasons we can't know but can imagine, or no one has managed to stay in academia long enough to reach that stage in their private lives. I find this new knowledge unexpected and rather discomforting.

## 2015

'Where are you from?'—'Ukraine.'—'Oh really? You don't look it!'— 'Eh...' [awkwardly]

# April 2015

I've been dispatched to represent my department in the organization committee of 'The EU and Emerging Powers,' a high-level biannual conference organized jointly by several Belgian universities. The final meeting before the conference has ended, and I am packing up my things to leave. The chair of the meeting approaches me and without any prelude declares elatedly: 'Oh, what's happening in Crimea! It's just like Kosovo and Alsace-Lorraine!' (not in those exact words but to that effect). I am astonished by this sudden fling of the topic at me (we've been talking about the EU, Brazil, and China for the past few hours and nothing alerted me to raise the thorns), by the indelicately light tone of the remark seeing as I am from Ukraine (he knows; that's precisely why he's raised the topic) and, most of all, by the comparison so dramatically false that I am shocked to hear it from a professor of political science. Caught totally off guard, I stand there, struggling to formulate a response that would simultaneously do justice to his severely misplaced statement, befit the discrepancy in status and otherwise perfectly amicable relationship between us, and not be too taxing on me emotionally. Or, in other words: how on Earth do I set him straight without exposing him, offending him, and getting too involved in this conversation?! To my own surprise, I reply detachedly,

'I am sorry, but your comparison is wrong on so many levels that I don't even know where to start and how not to offend you along the way. So let's not even go there.' Which, in turn, startles him. And—but of course!—he instantly retorts, 'Oh, I see you are very emotional about this. This must be a very emotional subject for you.' Yes, indeed, I get very emotional—that is: irritated, frustrated, outraged—by senior male professors flaunting incorrect statements, especially when it happens to be in my field of research! What was it again? 'Let me interrupt your expertise with my confidence.' There.

My direct response does make an impression, however: I get an email from him later that day apologizing and inviting me to talk about the situation in Ukraine in proper detail over lunch. He later invites me to contribute a chapter on the subject in his prospective book (which doesn't happen, but it's the thought that counts). We make peace.

## 2016

'Do you miss home?'—'Of course I do!' [Wait, are you subtly suggesting that this, here and now, is not my home, cannot be my home?..]

## July 2017

I arrive in Chengdu to teach in the University Immersion Program at Sichuan University. Bonnie, my assistant and savior for the two weeks of the summer school, glows with joy (and dare I suspect, pride) for being assigned, in her words, 'the youngest and the most beautiful Western professor.' One of the nights, she invites me to dine with her and her best friend, and as they sit opposite me, they repeatedly say how they admire my 'pretty narrow Western face with low cheekbones.' After a decade of being complemented in the West for my 'pretty round Eastern face with high cheekbones,' I find this remark simultaneously surprising and amusing. The thing is: in Ukraine, there are all sorts of faces, anywhere on the slim-to-round scale, and mine is just a face. My face.

One day after class, I am approached by Dmitri, a lecturer from Ekaterinburg who heard I was Ukrainian and is eager to discuss Russian atrocities in Crimea and in the East of Ukraine. ('How odd', I remember thinking then, 'for me to have to go all the way to China to meet—at last—a living Russian who admits we have a 'situation' and wants to talk about it!'). We agree to converse over dinner that evening, once the unbearable heat settles a little. At the end of the dinner, he insists on paying—even though we are roughly same age, same seniority, I am probably better off financially (seeing as I am based in Belgium, while he is based in Russia, and my trip will be fully reimbursed too), this meeting was our joint initiative and is *most certainly not* a date (and nothing in our conduct or conversation could have been taken to hint at one). Besides toxic Eastern European (or is it post-Soviet?) gender roles that require the man always pay—which he shares and I don't—there is absolutely no reason for him to pay. I protest, and we argue about it, balancing between politeness and firmness. It goes on and on, and, writing this now, I honestly don't remember who paid in the end.

## September 2017

I attend the Gender Mainstreaming Training (*sic*) for academic staff at our Faculty. There are exactly two men in the room and about 20 women, with me as the one foreigner. (Mind you: the gender ratio of permanent academic staff at the faculty is roughly the reverse, with not one female professor in my department at the time, and I am typically the only foreigner in the room). One of the two men has to be there due to his post within the Faculty and seizes the first opportunity to leave. The other one is genuinely interested in the subject and involved in the discussion, which he animates with honest questions 'from the other side,' unintimidated by being the only man in the training. Eventually, he admits that he only ever recruits male PhD students for considerations of doing fieldwork (when travel and sleep happen under imperfect conditions, so it is 'easier to be among guys') and also bonding (because 'you would not go for a beer after work with a female PhD student'—and what other ways to bond are there, really?!). He asks for our advice on whether and how he can get out of this pattern, and, besides the collective toned-down-furious 'just do it!', I remember one of the suggestions being trying out bonding over lunch or coffee-and-cake.

For the female participants, who could each deliver similar training themselves, it resembles a lousy group therapy session for frustrated women in academia.

## October 2017

Natalka, Kateryna, and I are finalizing the program for the closing conference of our *Civil Society in Post-Euromaidan Ukraine* project in Kyiv next month, with the special issue coming out in December. Only now does it strike us that ours unintentionally became an all-female project: we did select several contributions by male scholars following an open call for papers, but these dropped out along the way, and at this final stage it's only women on board. As we pause to reflect on this observation, three thoughts spring to my mind. An all-female project (with the majority based in or coming from the country)—'and yet' the outcome is a perfectly coherent, high-quality, timely product. Turns out there *are* women scholars out there, and *local* scholars on top of that! An all-female project—'and yet' we produced a special issue in one year from start to finish, despite many of us being primary caretakers for our children and some of us dealing with serious kids' illnesses, broken limbs, pregnancy loss, and even the unspeakable sorrow of child loss. Turns out women can and do deliver quality work on time, despite being immersed in the chaos of family life. An all-female project on civil society—'and yet' there are so many male scholars out there (holding most of the permanent positions, it appears). The vast majority of paper proposals we received came from women, and the few men we selected lost interest along the way—which makes one wonder about the gender allocation of research fields. I have a book title for a potential academic study on this: 'Men are from energy and security, women are from civil society and human rights.'

## 2018

'Are all Ukrainian women as strong and confident as you and talk as fast?'—'Eh...' [awkwardly]

## September 2018

Inspired by a workshop on critical ethnography, I embark on writing an autoethnographic essay on the superiority-inferiority dynamics in academia.[1] I quickly decide to write the essay as a diary, let the episodes speak for themselves and leave the reader to understand the points I am making 'to the best of their depravity,' as a Russian saying has it (and you are correct in thinking that this essay is written similarly). Brainstorming for the essay, I sketch out a few episodes that expose everyday sexism and gendered racism (and again you are correct in suspecting that several of those found their way into this piece).

I seriously doubt whether they rightfully belong in the essay, however, and as I write, this uneasiness grows. For one, I want my story to speak to—and for—the experiences of both male and female migrant academics, and so I believe I ought to make an honest attempt to tone gender down if I cannot keep it out altogether. More fundamentally: I don't want to speak of gender in an essay 'about inferiority complexes' because, well, I have never had an inferiority complex because of my gender, most certainly not in a professional context. Over-sexualization and over-feminization of women notwithstanding, *professionally* speaking, women in Ukraine are pretty emancipated—arguably more so and definitely longer so than women in the West. 'Long live communism!', I am afraid. My mother and aunties all had university education and careers; both my grannies had university education and careers; even my great-grandmothers had vocational training, and one of them worked as a 'village doctor' of sorts. I encountered the concept of 'stay-at-home-mom' in American period dramas about the 1950s, and it was not until I went to Western Europe and met my peers' mothers that I encountered actual stay-at-home-moms. The point is: growing up, nobody ever questioned my intellectual abilities or professional ambitions because of my gender. I was encouraged at every step and had endless role models within and without my family. 'Olya, know that you can be *anything* you want to be, *next to* being a wife and a mother.' (There's always a caveat, right?) I would object the dual burden and over-sexualization of women in society, I would, but it simply never occurred to me to feel inferior for being a woman. It was quite a cognitive dissonance, I must confess: coming to the 'advanced' West and discovering that 'housewife' was #1 career among women only a generation or two ago.

---

1     The essay was published as Olga Burlyuk, 'Fending off a triple inferiority complex in academia: An autoethnography', *Journal of Narrative Politics* 6/1 (2019): 28–50.

And so I delete all the 'gender episodes' from the draft. I don't so much as cut-and-paste them into another document for future reference: plain select-and-delete.

## 2019

'Do you miss home?'—'Of course I do!' [Wait, do locals ever get asked this question, or is it reserved for migrants?..]

## May 2019

I am in New York for the annual conference of the Association for the Study of Nationalities. It's the welcome reception, and as I gaze around the room, I catch myself speculating cynically what the odds are that the few women in bright-colored tight extravagant dresses and high-heeled shoes flew in directly from Central or Eastern Europe: 95 percent? 99? A full 100? I notice it; everyone notices it; and, to be sure, it is *actually* discussed in one of the circles of people I find myself in at some point during the evening. The thing is: I know not to read absolutely anything about a woman's intelligence or morality from her clothes. But I know that others do. And it drives me mad.

As an Eastern European woman in the West, you find yourself—I find myself—in a paradoxical position: it is expected that you dress up, and when you do, you become a topic of conversation and occasionally a laughing stock, too. As soon as you figure that out, you feel compelled to dress down, to 'mimic the walls' as my mother calls it. And then you come to realize that this is also expected of you: it is considered *only normal* for you to want to conceal your Eastern Europeanness—to take it off, quite literally—and blend in. So much so that eventually you feel compelled to dress up as a form of protest. It is a Sophie's choice, really, with no outcome preferable over the other. Because what you want is simply to dress as you feel like waking up that day; but, no matter what you go for, people will read something 'typically Eastern European' into it, and usually not in your favor.

So there I stand at the conference venue, listening to the enthusiastic chatter about a woman's dress, in my navy blue formal pants, a dark blue silk blouse (with a bold flower pattern and ruffled cuffs, however!), low-heeled black shoes, a deliberately modest jewelry set, make-up 'au naturel', hair pinned back. In other words: meticulously censored, my inner protest screaming silently through the ruffled cuffs. Looking appropriate-with-a-twist, seemingly intelligent, somewhat European, almost Western (never mind the cheekbones). One foot here, one foot there. Neither here, nor there. Tired and resentful.

I go to the MET Opera later that night, and when the guy sitting next to me asks 'where are you from?' and I reply 'take a guess', he pauses a moment and says... 'European undefined.' A mic drop.

## October 2019

I arrive at a work meeting, and before it commences formally, someone starts gossiping about a suspected affair between a PhD student, a beautiful young Eastern European woman based in Western Europe, and a senior professor, a proverbial 'old white Western European man.' This is the first I have heard of it, although I know both parties personally. So I just sit there and listen, confused as to whether I am startled more by the very idea of an affair between these two (heh?!) or by the sheer fact that we are having a conversation about it (huh?!). The matter is discussed enthusiastically, with a mixture of curiosity, amusement, puzzlement, and disapproval. The people are setting the facts straight (who-saw-what-when and how this all adds up or doesn't), checking these against the girl's supposed relationship status ('I thought she had a boyfriend, no?') and purity of character—and concluding that, if true, this is one inappropriate situation. I feel extremely uncomfortable throughout, but I cannot pin down in that moment what about this discussion *specifically* puts me off—besides the fact that we are having it, obviously—so I do not intervene.

It hits me later what it was (I cannot let go and mull over this for days): not a word of judgement, or appraisal to that effect, was said about *the guy*. The one of the two who is much older. Who is way more senior professionally. Who is 'a Westerner.' Who is most likely married. And who is most certainly taking advantage of his social and legal status—and her lack thereof. Yet there were six of us in that room: three men and three women. If anything, the conversation should have been about how appalled we all were with the apparent abuse of power by the proverbial *old white man*. As this realization dawns on me, I am sincerely stunned that it took me days to articulate an observation *this obvious*, to spot an elephant-in-the-room *that big*. And that no one else did. What does that say about each of us separately and as a group? I also wonder to what extent the entertaining overtone of the discussion was due to the fact that the girl was Eastern European—and so the whole situation somehow, consciously or subconsciously, simply 'fit the bill.' Would we be having a similar conversation if the 'she' in the story was, say, German or Danish? Would we be similarly blind to the elephant in the room? Finally, I question myself about how far my own 'temporary analytical paralysis' during the conversation and after was because I was Eastern European myself, the only one in that room. Did my brain go into some kind of freeze-mode to evade 'tarnishing by association' or what?

I feel at once sad and furious. Silence gives consent, the saying goes, and I ought to revoke mine. I consider writing an email to the people in that meeting, pointing at the elephant, but I decide to raise the issue in person at our next meeting instead. I don't, however, as I cannot come up with an elegant way to do so and imagine it to be extremely confrontational and awkward, too.

Silence gives consent.

## 2020

'Do you miss home?'—'Of course I miss Ukraine, if that's what you are asking. I miss my family, my friends, my favorite foods and places.' [And I won't tell you that I can no longer tell where home is. Perhaps there can be several? Or perhaps there is no such place?...]

## February 2020

I am invited to speak about my autoethnography on inferiority and superiority in academia at the EDGE seminar at the Free University of Brussels (VUB). Vjosa—who suggested EDGE invite me—and I decide to frame the talk as a conversation, and we check in the day before to synchronize on what and how. Incidentally, we realize that both of us plan on wearing formal black dresses (only hers will be a trendy little black dress and mine will be a maternity one, as I am eight months pregnant at the time). We jokingly conspire that Vjosa should wear a bright red lipstick to the talk, and I should apply blue eyeshadow: to pay tribute to our Balkan and Eastern European roots, respectively. 'Consider it an intervention on the Western aesthetics!', she says, and we laugh. The blue eyeshadow is too much for me, though, and does not go with the black dress at all, so I apply grey eyeshadow instead. I paint my nails red to compensate.

And so I sit at the event: a pregnant Ukrainian woman who thinks. A Ukrainian woman who thinks. A woman who thinks. A woman.

# Works cited

Sara Ahmed, *Living a Feminist Life* (Duke University Press, 2017). https://doi.org/10.1215/9780822373377

Olga Burlyuk, 'Fending off a triple inferiority complex in academia: An autoethnography', *Journal of Narrative Politics* 6/1 (2019): 28–50.

Irena Karpa, *Yak Vyhodyty Zamizh Stilky Raziv, Skilky Zahochete* [How to marry as many times as you want] (#knyholav, 2020).

# EMBODIED DIFFERENCES AND (NON) WHITENESS

# 18. Wiping the Smudge off the Window: The Darkest Time as a Student in Europe

*Lydia Namatende-Sakwa*

## To Manchester, I come!

The much-coveted scholarship to pursue my PhD at a university in Manchester within the United Kingdom had come with so much excitement for a Ugandan woman like me. It was not going to be easy—I knew that. My baby Gail was only 2.5 months old—yes, a breast-feeding, white-eyed, black-haired, beautiful baby girl—and my other two children (George and Gaby) were 4 and 2 years old. While I would have loved them to come with me, my funding was nowhere near enough to support a family. How was I going to do this? I occasionally asked myself. Matters were made worse by what I referred to as 'tales of damnation' regarding leaving my young family. These tales started right after I announced that I had received a scholarship to pursue my PhD abroad.

I remember bumping into a friend and former classmate at a supermarket. She cautioned me about leaving my baby, stating, 'Lydia, you know your baby needs you.' Another male colleague, who had previously left his wife and children to pursue a doctorate, warned: "You will regret this!" And another female colleague at work assured me that: 'Your baby will never bond with you.' I struggled with these voices in my head—reasoning with myself that children need us all of the time. When I was in that labor ward as a 27-year-old having my first baby, I

    https://doi.org/10.11647/OBP.0331.18

had yearned for my late mother. I consoled myself that, in fact, children never stop needing their mothers. With reassurances and support from Andrew, my husband, coupled with the anticipated bright future that a PhD from Europe promised, I set off for my maiden journey to Europe.

At Heathrow, I came to the realization that I was "different" when, in the immigration queue, I was the only one interrogated for the lengthiest of time. What I thought was routine questioning eventually raised my brow when it went on and on as other passengers flocked past me. The immigration officer asked, amidst other questions, why I looked different in my passport picture than I did in person: I wondered, in retrospect, whether he had asked the other passengers that question? At that time, I politely replied that in the passport photo, I had had shorter hair, which I had re-grown.

Having made accommodation arrangements from a listing posted by a student for a student-share apartment, I made it to the post office where I was to meet my roommate, who had described what she would be wearing, as had I. Standing in the winter cold, which I was experiencing for the very first time as winter darkness also started to dawn, I recurrently called my 'roommate,' until the phone was switched off. I could no longer reach her. In hindsight—in my mind's eye—I could swear that I saw someone fitting her description pass by. Perhaps, as I thought months later, she had seen a black me and decided against sharing accommodation with me. It was now time to check in with the other accommodation contact made while in Uganda. I received directions to the apartment. At that point, my fingers, which had to drag the suitcase with all my possessions, were numb, as were my feet, which had to walk about eight kilometer to the apartment. I cried all the way there. Hungry. Cold. Distraught.

After ringing the doorbell, the door was opened to show my potential roommates, about five all-white young women, who dismissively said half-hearted 'hellos' before continuing with a hearty conversation over dinner. One of them showed me to my room, which was alone on the top floor. I dragged my suitcase up the stairs, hoping I would get a breather. Nothing could have prepared me for the closet-sized room with neither a wardrobe nor space for a study table and chair. As I sat on the bed with tears rolling down my face, I heard the vibration of the room as someone adjacent flushed the toilet. I knew then that I would not make compromises with my accommodation. On calling the landlady to negotiate for a short stay, she firmly asked me to either take the room and sign the contract or leave right away. This was a difficult option given the winter pitch-blackness at about 7:00 pm, in a strange country. I sat at the stairs—tears seamlessly rolling down my cheeks.

In explaining my dilemma, one of the girls talked to the landlady, who then allowed me to stay for an exorbitant 60 pounds a night. This was, nonetheless, such a relief. In what I thought was empathy for me, one of the girls asked me to help myself to some food in the kitchen as they all stepped out of the apartment, seemingly to go out. I really appreciated this. Little did I know that the food had been offered only out of politeness—empty dinner dishes were stacked in the kitchen sink. This was the opening to the darkest time in my life, accentuated by my meeting with Prof. Karen Hunters (not her real name), my PhD supervisor—whom I focus this narrative on.

## My supervisor: Damned if I did—damned still if I didn't!

After settling into accommodation with an Indian couple from whom I rented a room, I prepared for a meeting with Karen and, subsequently, Lianka Barington (not her real name either), my second supervisor. Waiting my turn outside her office, I saw Karen engage with someone I later learned was one of her favorite PhD students. There was laughter and positive energy, which I looked forward to partaking in. To my surprise, the expression on Karen's face immediately changed to a stern animosity as soon as I stepped into the room. This was the marker of my supervisory meetings with Karen, who, as I came to realize, did not believe in my potential to undertake a PhD program in this prestigious school. I was damned as far as Karen was concerned: damned if my work was great—when she declared doubts I had done it myself, leading to a barrage of questions which I responded to with reassurances that, indeed, it was *my* work—but also damned if the work was not great, when she suggested that the university's standards were too high for me! In one supervisory meeting, as I presented my work, Karen burst out laughing—I have never known why. Lianka (my second supervisor) and I waited for her to finish her raucous laugh before I proceeded with my presentation.

Karen, as I later learnt from one of my lecturers at the University, had strongly advocated for that scholarship to be awarded to a home rather than an international student. Losing to the majority on the award panel, the scholarship was awarded to an international student— who happened to be me. Given her expertise in gender studies/feminist work, which underpinned my PhD proposal, Karen was chosen as my supervisor. Was this an opportunity for her to disprove the panel? To demonstrate that as an international student I was not worthy of this award? That I was not academically astute enough?

The precarity I felt at school was accentuated when conversations with classmates about my zip code revealed that Rasholm, where I lived in a beautiful house, was actually an unsafe part of Manchester! I remember having heard what I thought were gunshots in the night and having dived off my bed to read on the floor, averting the risk of possible stray bullets. When I did eventually ask my housemates about these shots, they reassured me that it was, in fact, fireworks, which I had believed until friends from the Ugandan community cast doubt on this tale. This meant that I had to leave campus early, walking home in fear of the unknown. This further messed with my peace.

## Christmas holidays: Returning home

My light in the tunnel was the imminent Christmas holiday when I would return home to visit my family in Uganda. The five months away from my children and husband had been the toughest time—emotionally draining. I had left a breast-feeding baby Gail, whom I 'heard' cry from time to time all the way from Uganda. I sometimes cried myself to sleep—cried over the phone as my helpless husband tried to comfort the inconsolable me, who questioned my sacrifices in the quest for a PhD, which had started to look elusive—a chasing of the wind.

When Christmas break finally came, I could not fathom what it would feel like to hold my baby—and my other two children. Gail, a most peaceful baby, accustomed to her nanny and father, pulled away when this 'stranger' excitedly tried to hold her. I had to give her at least a week to peep at me from a distance. She eventually ran and sat on my lap and then ran away again until the day when she finally settled on my lap and comfortably let me hold her to sleep. I took a much-needed two-month-long holiday, bonding with my family—dreading all the while that I would have to leave them. At the end of the holiday, I stayed an extra two weeks, which in the end, cost me the renewal of my scholarship.

## 'Will you come back soon?' On returning to the UK

I returned to the UK broken—my son had looked me in the eye at the airport, and with a dimpled cheek, he had asked me: 'Will you come back soon?' and I had replied, 'Yes! Yes, I will!' I got onto the plane in tears. Little did I know that these tears were but a drop in the ocean compared to the ones I would cry on my way out of the UK in pain and humiliation.

I returned to a supervisor—Karen—who was up in arms that I had stayed longer, even if I had communicated that I had not been well. This culminated in a battle in which I fought tooth and nail to get back into her "good" graces—in vain. The progress reports she had written in the six months I had been at the school had cast doubt on my ability to pursue the PhD program. The magnitude of my stress culminated in illness for which I was hospitalized. While Lianka visited and brought me some books to keep me occupied in the hospital, I only bumped into Karen at the university, who commented about my physical appearance stating, 'You have lost so much weight! You look too thin for a person who is not thin!'

At the height of tension between Karen and I, one of the administrators advised that I apply for a change of supervisor. I rejected this proposal with confidence that, since I was a hardworking student, Karen would come around. This was the biggest mistake I made during this journey as we continued in a turbulent supervisory relationship. In the end, Karen was required to recommend me for the renewal of my scholarship. She tossed me back and forth until she eventually and grudgingly wrote a recommendation, after so much begging and fretting on my part. My scholarship was not renewed, and after a gruesome semester punctuated with worry and stress, I returned home—burning with shame—shame that I would be looked at as a failure—shame that I had left my children—only to chase the wind—shame. Shame. Shame. I picked up the pieces—with the help of my husband and my dad. I stumbled up—tried to find my feet. Dad reassured me that 'destiny can be paused, but it cannot be stopped!' I held on to this.

Now that my funding had been pulled out from under my feet, I had to downgrade from the PhD to an MSc, which required me to write a dissertation. Karen and Lianka supervised my dissertation. Karen specifically commended the 'hard work' and 'a really good analysis' as Lianka complimented 'the breadth and depth' of my reading. I submitted my dissertation and wiped what I thought were the dwindling tears of the darkest time. I refocused on searching for funding to do the PhD with the strength that the MSc from Manchester would be a vantage point for the application for PhD funding. Nothing could have prepared me for the 58% on my provisional transcript. This was below the 60% pass mark for dissertations at the University at the time. I received another shocker when I discovered that Karen was one of the markers. I knew (as I know now) that Karen had used this opportunity to prove the point that I was incapable of doing a PhD—a point that dominated all the progress reports she had written about me. I questioned why Karen had given positively flattering feedback only to grade the dissertation below the pass mark. I consulted Lianka, who was shocked by the outcome and by the fact that she had not been asked to second-mark the dissertation.

## Fighting a losing battle

It was now time to throw my PhD plans out the window—at least momentarily—and to fight a losing battle against a professor whose colleagues *daren't* oppose. And yes, my battle was public knowledge in the department 'corridors'. Indeed, three classmates with whom I had not shared my story had reached out using email, empathizing with me and encouraging me to seek a re-mark. Two of them stated that they had heard about my conundrum from their own supervisors.

When I applied for a re-mark, Karen fought tooth and nail to block it. Karen was a professor and one of the most senior colleagues, even in terms of age. In hindsight, I question whether her colleagues could have dared challenge her? What would it have meant to re-mark and/or challenge the position of a senior colleague? Would they have dared overturn her decision? What would that have meant for collegiality and/or the school reputation?

The 58% mark was two marks short of the cut-off to continue with the PhD. Karen, who had provided affirmative feedback during the writing of the dissertation, had deliberately sabotaged any chances of continuation at the university when she had the chance to mark the book. I questioned why she had vehemently, in letters and emails back and forth, blocked a re-mark if she had assessed me objectively and had nothing to hide. This question has remained with me since. In hindsight, I was but a black smudge on her white wall—and wipe me out she did.

## 'Destiny can be paused. But it cannot be stopped!'

With reassurance from Lianka about the quality of my dissertation, we co-authored an article, which was immediately accepted and published in one of the most highly rated journals in my field of research. And, holding on to the words of wisdom from my father about destiny, I rubbed the dust off from this fall, resolving to look for funding again. I was admitted first into Ghent University in Belgium under the university's Extraordinary Research Fund (BOF) scholarship. I worked with an amazing supervisor—Prof. Chia Longman—in pursuing a PhD in gender and diversity. I was also admitted to the doctorate in curriculum and teaching as a Fulbright Scholar at Teachers College Columbia University, an Ivy League School in New York, where I worked under a magnificent professor, Nancy Lesko. I pursued these programs in different disciplines and contexts concurrently, graduating with two doctoral degrees in November 2016 and May 2017, respectively. As expressed in the title of William Shakespeare's play published in 1623, *All's well that ends well.*

Still, I carry Karen with me—flashes of her come and go. One of those moments inspired a poem.

> A Black Smudge off the Window
> Wiping the smudge off the window
> Is what you did, What you did to me.
> Wiping the smudge off the window,
> Was not enough.
> Not enough for you.
> You had to dig,
> Dig the deepest hole.
> You had to bury the smudge,
> Bury me to leave no trace.
> —Lydia, 21 November 2012

# 19. A Letter to Future Adoptee Researchers: On Being a Researcher of Color in Belgium

*Atamhi Cawayu*

This letter started as an essay to share my reflections as a racialized researcher in white Belgian academia. However, I did not feel comfortable producing another essay that followed the conventions of the Ivory Tower, especially since this edited volume welcomed other creative forms of written texts. I decided to transform my essay into a letter to future adoptee researchers, hopefully offering room for dialogue with the reader.

## Dear future adoptee researcher

How great that you are interested in pursuing an academic career by examining transnational adoption. I am happy to share some of my personal experiences of being an adoptee researcher employed in a white institution. Since I am in the final months of my doctoral studies, this allows me to reflect honestly on my own doctoral journey. It has certainly been filled with ups and downs, with feelings of loneliness and togetherness, and emotions of disillusion and happiness. I assume that these feelings and emotions are part of the doctoral trajectory at large and are also present in fellow non-adopted researchers' academic journeys. Nevertheless, with this letter I would like to elaborate on my academic journey as a politically engaged researcher of color in Belgian academia and demonstrate how activism and research can be

    https://doi.org/10.11647/OBP.0331.19

compatible. As we live the reality of being removed from our parents, community, and land, we do not want to examine this topic in a sterile way but instead contribute to processes of social change and turn the narrative on transnational adoption.

## From orphan to activist, from activist to researcher

It is not so strange to research a topic that is very close to your heart. Nonetheless, during your academic journey, you will often hear from strangers that your adoption background might prevent you from conducting objective scientific research. They will tell you that you are too subjective, too biased, too critical, too involved, too everything because you will never be able to comply with their standards. For those criticasters, our adoption histories are seen as a disadvantage, while white non-adopted researchers are often seen as the embodiment of objectivity. Yet, I consider adoptee's voices as indispensable in adoption research. Studying adoption without adoptee researchers is like studying women without female researchers or studying migrants without migrant researchers. We are the ones who live it. We are the ones who stayed short or long term in orphanages. We are the ones that lost all legal ties with our families of origin. We are the ones that have been relocated and displaced from one continent to another. We are the ones whose names were changed. We are the ones that were assigned to white strangers that spoke a language we did not understand but we had to call them 'family.' We do have the lived experience of being adopted, and I rather see this as an advantage instead of a disadvantage. Feminist methodologies provide us with methodological tools and concepts, such as positionality and reflexivity, that allow us to share our personal involvement with the topic and how this is present in the research process. Fortunately, the field of adoption studies has been transformed over the years. The first generation of adoptee researchers has paved the way for the newer generations, including myself. I am very glad to notice that more adoptee researchers are entering the academic field of transnational adoption. That said, I think we have come to the part where I explain my own personal journey of becoming a researcher, and what my motivations to start doctoral studies and examine transnational adoption were.

I was born in the indigenous city of El Alto (Bolivia) in October 1992, and was adopted six months later by a white Belgian working-class couple. I had a happy childhood and a lovely adoptive family. Only after my first trip back to Bolivia did I realize that my adoption did not only 'give' but it also 'took' many things from me. I searched for other Bolivian adoptees in Belgium and became acquainted with a fellow Bolivian adoptee, who was also adopted the same year and month, with the difference being that her adoption was an illegal one. I returned to Bolivia to obtain more information about my pre-adoptive past, but was confronted with institutional issues. According to Bolivian law, my adoption did not happen, as the respective adoption intermediaries did not finalize the adoption process in Bolivia, which means that I am registered as an 'orphan' to this day. In addition, I discovered that my orphanage was hiding parts of my adoption documents. Needless to say, the return trip was a disillusioning experience.

I started to develop a critical stance towards the global system of transnational adoption. Fueled by the injustices present in the current adoption system, I became politically engaged in the public adoption debate in Belgium and participated in political hearings in the Flemish Parliament. At the same time, I decided to write my second Master's thesis in gender and diversity on the lived experiences of Bolivian adoptees in Flanders. The field of critical adoption studies not only enhanced my academic knowledge of transnational adoption but also helped me develop a substantiated vision that I deployed in my adoptee activism. After graduating, I wanted to pursue a professional career in the field of adoption. Eventually, I was hired as a staff member at the Flemish Central Authority for Adoption, a governmental institution that supervises transnational adoption practices. This work experience gave me a behind-the-scenes view of adoption practices and nuanced my understanding by giving me insights into how adoption policies came about and who has responsibility for them. At the same time, I was also working on a proposal to conduct research on transnational adoption, with specific attention to the families of origin and stakeholders in the adoption system in Bolivia. The idea of doing research on this came from my own questions and interests at the time, as someone without any information available on my family of origin.

Nevertheless, I wanted to understand other families' stories of relinquishment and adoption. I wanted to understand the social, cultural, political, and economic circumstances that led to child relinquishment in Bolivia. I wanted to understand why thousands of Bolivian/indigenous children were displaced and relocated to families in the Global North. In addition, my experiences in my activist work made me realize that, despite my knowledge of the theme, I would always be considered as an 'adoptee' instead of an 'expert.' Whilst an academic career would provide me with the skills and tools to conduct a thorough investigation, this is not always a guarantee of being considered an 'expert.' For others, our personal stories will always be more interesting than our academic expertise on the theme. Nonetheless, I chose the academic route so that I could contribute to the democratization of academic knowledge on adoption. My involvement in adoptee organizations on the one hand, and my previous work experience at the Central Authority on the other hand, motivated me to bridge academia and the adoption field. To my great surprise, my research proposal was accepted. It was like a dream come true, but little did I know that the academic world would not turn out to be the safe space I had thought it would be.

## Surviving white academia

Let us imagine you have made it into academia. Then what? Academia may seem like a safe space that is open to new insights and critical perspectives; one which celebrates diversity. This might be true to some extent. However, I consider academia an elitist institution that upholds the same structural inequalities of race, gender, and class as the rest of society. If you are not part of academia, this might sound very abstract, but I hope to provide some examples throughout this letter. The last thing I want to do is discourage anyone from pursuing their academic dreams, especially because there are too few researchers of color. The higher you go on the academic ladder, the whiter and more masculine it becomes. There is a great need for researchers with all kinds of different backgrounds to diversify the academy and challenge the status quo of those who possess institutional power.

In retrospect, I would say I started my academic journey with a large portion of naïveté. I recall my first day as a doctoral student at Ghent

University very well. In the early morning, I had an appointment with my supervisor to discuss what I would focus on in the first weeks of my academic career. Then I went to my new workspace, which I shared with a fellow doctoral student. The office was still fairly empty, a bit uninviting, and looked somewhat industrial. Despite that, I felt really happy that I finally had the time to read all the books and articles that were on my reading list. The research center I was affiliated with supported critical, feminist, and anthropological research, and this allowed me to focus on theories and methodologies that really spoke to me. I decided to immerse myself in postcolonial and decolonial thought and critical methodologies that provided me with tools for social change. During my first year as a doctoral student, I was very enthusiastic about participating in seminars, conferences, and courses on a range of topics. I was very eager to learn, expand my horizons, and become familiar with new theoretical insights and concepts. In the beginning, I considered these events interesting and challenging, but later I started to get disappointed when I saw how, for the umpteenth time, a prominent white scholar's theoretical framework was applied to anthropological research. The academic space slowly began to disenchant me. Do not get me wrong, I believe all academics can make a valuable contribution, regardless of their race. However, using Pierre Bourdieu as a central theoretical framework to analyze the daily life practices in a village in South Asia and not mentioning one South Asian author sounds problematic. I noticed how Northern theories and concepts were constantly reproduced by (white) European academics during several seminars and conferences. This made me even more interested in the knowledge production of scholars in the Global South. I learned about Southern theories, feminisms, and methodologies. The fact that my research topic was situated in Bolivia undoubtedly played a role in my curiosity about Southern and marginalized epistemologies.

Then comes the question, 'What do you do when you consider certain approaches, theories, and concepts used in academic research ethically problematic?' Although most seminars are considered spaces of exchange and feedback, I sometimes felt a certain fragility when pointing out the Eurocentrism in the research presented. Similar to this, I also noticed that when I addressed people about everyday words and phrases with racial connotations—for example, the Dutch expression 'a

Chinese volunteer' (an expression used for someone who is forced to volunteer)—I felt some kind of resistance and even negation. I think we all have our blind spots when it comes to topics such as race, gender, age, disability, and so on. Nevertheless, I naïvely thought that fellow social scientists would be open to a constructive conversation, but instead, I often returned home empty-handed. This had the effect that I started to withdraw from certain activities, seminars, and meetings. I did not feel comfortable anymore, and I did not have the energy to raise these issues again. Writing a doctoral dissertation was already challenging enough for me, and I preferred to focus on my academic work and adoptee activism. Fortunately, I had other colleagues of color with whom I could reflect extensively during breaks or after working hours on dealing with racial issues in academia and sharing experiences. I am eternally grateful to the Belgian-Nepalese researcher, Hari Prasad Adhikari Sacré, who has been there for me during almost my whole doctoral journey. Together, we organized back in 2019 an event called 'Surviving White Institutions,' in which we invited scholars and professionals of color to reflect collectively on working in white institutional spaces. This event led to new connections and gave me the energy to continue in white academia.

## The rise of adoptee researchers

Maybe some good news: I can reassure you that adoptee researchers are on the rise. It has not always been like that. Back in the early 2000s, the first generation of adoptee researchers entered the academic field of adoption. At that time, the perspectives of transnational adoptees were largely absent, and the field was dominated by white non-adopted academics. The influential book *Outsiders Within: Writing on Transracial Adoption* (Trenka, Oparah, and Shin, 2006), composed by adoptee authors, aimed to rewrite the dominant adoption narratives through the contributions of predominantly adoptee scholars, adoptee authors, adoptee activists, and adoptee artists. In the introduction, they note that mainly white academics, professionals, and adoptive parents dominated the literature on transnational adoption in the previous decades. Their book has been influential in providing artistic, scholarly, and literary counternarratives to transnational adoption. I have great admiration and respect for these first-generation adoptee authors who paved the way for newer generations of adoptee scholars. This also means that adoptee researchers are no longer marginalized in the field of critical adoption studies, but have contributed substantially to transforming the field. Yet that does not mean that the field is dominated by us. There are still more non-adopted researchers than adoptee researchers. And even though I greatly admire both for their work, I remain a bit skeptical of white non-adopted academics that decide to research us, interview us, analyze us, apply their Eurocentric concepts to our stories, sometimes misinterpret us, and talk about us at conferences that most of us adoptees cannot attend due to the high conference fee or the closed nature, which upholds academic elitism—some exceptions notwithstanding.

When I entered academia, I wanted to disseminate the knowledge produced within critical adoption studies to professionals, stakeholders, and directly impacted people. Because of my background as an activist in adoptee communities and as a professional in the adoption sector, I wanted to bridge these different areas and stir up a constructive dialogue between all parties. Together with my supervisor and other scholars and professionals, we decided to organize a symposium, which later received the name *Symposium Intercountry Adoption: How to Continue? Perspectives from the Social Sciences and Humanities*. In contrast to many academic adoption conferences, in this one, adoptees played a leading role either as academics, professionals, or by sharing their own experiences. The symposium was well-received by the adoptee participants, but less so by the adoption agencies—probably because the symposium did not shy away from addressing the abuses and illegalities inherent in transnational adoption in past and current practices.

As a result, a debriefing was organized by the Flemish Central Authority to engage in dialogue with the adoption agencies. Instead of having a constructive conversation, the professionals from the adoption agencies critiqued the research outcomes of several academic presentations. They said the empirical data was 'dated,', 'not generalizable,' 'too biased,' and were unwilling to engage with the suggested recommendations. At that point, I realized that, despite my efforts to engage adoption agencies in an open dialogue, they would never accept research findings that exposed the flaws in the global adoption system and its vulnerability to potential abuses and malpractices. It was the wake-up call that I needed because for too long I naïvely thought that my research would contribute to a social change in the adoption field, but I realized then that my research would possibly be put aside and read as 'too subjective.' This all made me wonder for whom I was making all these efforts, especially when professionals working in the adoption system did not want to consider research outcomes. To be honest, I had an existential crisis during that time, and I questioned the added value of my own research if nothing would be done with it anyway. It saddened me deeply knowing that the adoption agencies responsible for abuses and malpractices did not want to take any responsibility. Instead, they minimized these issues and emphasized the positive outcomes that come along with adoption—as if positive adoption stories erase the lived experiences of adoptees who have been kidnapped, trafficked, and sold to the industry of transnational adoption.

## Pursue your dreams, we are the change

I hope this letter did not discourage you from writing that research proposal. Never give up on your dreams and keep following your ambitions. I realize I have focused too much on the challenges of being an adoptee researcher of color in academia, but I have also had many beautiful moments. My doctoral journey has introduced me to some wonderful people, critical minds, and excellent scholars. I greatly appreciate the relationships I have been able to build with Bolivian adoptees, first families, and adoptive families I have met through my research project and who have let me into their lives. Furthermore, my research has allowed me to stay for long-term periods in Bolivia, which not only let me familiarize myself with the field of child protection and adoption, but also permitted me to build lasting relationships with people I encountered along the way.

Despite the disillusionments during my doctoral studies—and thanks to the happy moments—I have not given up yet. Academia allowed me to engage with critical scholarship and to organize numerous small-scale events open to academics and non-academics. I strongly believe that knowledge should not be confined to the academic world, but that exchanges, dialogues, and open conversations are necessary if we want to continue the transformative process of knowledge exchange.

In addition, I have lost my naïveté about academia, and my doctoral dissertation no longer intends to radically transform the adoption sector. I am now writing the thesis primarily for myself and for the Bolivian adoptee community. That said, I am convinced that social change will happen, partly through us and our work; this has already started happening. In recent years, I have seen an increase in the number of students expressing their dissatisfaction with the curriculum as it is too white and Eurocentric. On top of that, more student organizations and movements are organizing actions to decolonize the university. In the field of adoption, I have seen some changes over the seven years I have been actively involved. Adoptee voices are much more present now than in the past. On the political level, the global adoption system is questioned much more than before, and several European governments have installed commissions to examine abuses in the past and current adoption system. All this shows me that, over a period of several years, critical voices still seeped through. Someday the world will look different thanks to all our small efforts.

If you have any more questions or doubts, feel free to contact me. I am not sure if I will still be in academia then but let us see what the future holds for me.

With Love,
Atamhi Cawayu

# 20. Inside the Migrant Academic's Body: Strategic Outsider within Toxic Substructures

## Sama Khosravi Ooryad

Black and Third World people are expected to educate white people as to our humanity. Women are expected to educate men. Lesbians and gay men are expected to educate the heterosexual world. The oppressors maintain their position and evade their responsibility for their own actions. There is a constant drain of energy in redefining ourselves and devising realistic scenarios for altering the present and constructing the future.

Audre Lorde, *Sister Outsider: Essays and Speeches* (1984), p. 115

Our task is to remember the power and significance of our words; like when Audre told us that we weren't meant to survive (and yet here we are), or when June reminded us that we are the ones we have been waiting for. It's up to us to shift the ways that we care for each other and ourselves within institutions that are designed to exploit our contributions and use our bodies to fill their diversity quotas. We must work to create a new paradigm of 'normal' that is rooted in vitality instead of stress if we are to make it through the academy and live to tell our stories.

Analena Hope, *Can I Live?* (2012), par. 7

What is it like to be an outsider? How does it feel to be slapped in the face by numerous subtle yet toxic moments from every direction—to constantly hit 'brick walls'? These are certainly not easy questions, and they have no straightforward answers. They evoke an archive of pain and suffering, as well as countless moments of exclusion within and beyond academic spaces. These feelings can only be expressed by those

 https://doi.org/10.11647/OBP.0331.20

who experience them: people of color, queer communities, religious and ethnic minorities, and individuals from the Global South. These groups are 'outsiders' to history and society; yet moments of exclusion persist and are felt by many people who do not fit the dominant norms.

One principal site of power in which such exclusionary practices continue to be implicitly or explicitly prevalent is (Western) academia. Still, there should be lines of flight and holes to drill into the solid form of power from within the aura of rigidity that such institutions (and their practitioners) impose on 'outsiders.' How can one remain part of a hierarchical institution—in this case, academia—and assume the positionality of an outsider? Who is an outsider? And what could help them contest the power structures? How can we curse the power and remain 'outside' while still forming coalitions?

After I joined the gender studies program at Utrecht University in September 2017, I experienced an incident that may appear trivial but, to me, was eye-opening. I had received the prestigious Erasmus Mundus scholarship to study women's and gender studies in Europe at two European universities as part of the GEMMA Master's degree program (an EU-funded Erasmus Mundus Master's in women's and gender studies in Europe). GEMMA is a postgraduate programme that consists of two years of study at two chosen centers out of seven European universities that participate in the consortium. The program offers fully funded scholarships to non-EU students. Scholarship recipients in this program are mainly from developing or underprivileged countries. As both a non-European student coming from 'outside' of Europe and a scholarship holder, I felt responsible and grateful for the opportunity. I had heard about the renowned gender studies program at Utrecht University, and I was elated to pursue my MA there.

Shortly after the courses started, I received an email from two Dutch classmates containing an invitation to a party-discussion for students of the university's gender studies research Master's program. Such events involved friendly discussion circles around gender issues outside of a classroom format. The only part of the invitation that caught my attention was a statement at the end of the email where my classmates clarified that *only* RMA (Research Master's) students were welcome. Upon reading the word '*only*,' which is italicized here for emphasis, I, as a GEMMA student who was part of the same class, felt immediately excluded from that community. It implied that GEMMA students are not gender studies students and ignored the fact that we were also conducting research and taking part in classes. Later, I shared my thoughts about the word *'only'* with one of my teachers, who offered a justification of the incident. Eventually, I concluded that the incident was not as problematic as I had initially assumed.

As the course continued, I totally forgot about that little word: *only*. Nevertheless, it had a subconscious effect on me over time. I began to feel an invisible wall take shape within me regarding these three letters: RMA. Notably, I was not the only GEMMA student in the class; there were others, some of whom were from other European countries, though they were not (full) scholarship holders. Most of us who had come from outside of Europe (that is, the EU) were receiving scholarships as GEMMA students. However, over the course of my studies, I realized that the clear-cut divide between GEMMA students (and all scholarship holders) and the regular RMA students was not simply a matter of naming or cross-institutional lining, but in fact a result of the invisible 'brick wall' (Ahmed, 2017) built from many *only* moments. Thus, it was an intersectional issue that, at least to me, differentiated between those who had enough money to pay the expensive Dutch tuition fees and those who did not, those who were European and did not encounter numerous multiple difficulties while studying, and those who were non-European and had to confront such challenges—in short, between the privileged and the underprivileged. Yet, because some of the GEMMA students received 'money,' we were still perceived as somehow in a better situation than those who might have to work during their studies. This mindset seemed unfair to me, as I and my fellow scholarship holders could not have afforded to come to Europe in the first place without such a scholarship. As a woman with minimal savings after years of working on my own in Iran's cruel capital of Tehran, I did not have the luxury of coming to Europe to study as a self-funded student. Thus, for me, the three letters 'RMA' gradually came to represent privilege, whiteness, and wealthiness, while 'GEMMA' became equivalent to being non-wealthy, people of color, and so on.

In her classical article *Learning From the Outsider Within: The Sociological Significance of Black Feminist Thought* (1986), Patricia Hill Collins discusses how the marginal and outsider position of African American scholars in academia have endowed them with creativity and practical insights that remain overlooked by their white male colleagues.

She uses the term 'outsider within' to describe the marginal but creative position of Black feminist thought (Hill Collins, 1986, 15). On this basis, Hill Collins elaborates on how Black feminist thought, as an 'outsider' in academia, offers practical potential for conducting innovative research. She posits that outsiders, such as women of color, are especially attentive to the interconnected notions of race, class, and gender, for example, and are thus highly conscious of racial, class, and gender-related patterns in performing research; by comparison, white 'insiders' in academia may hardly recognize the same patterns. An outsider within is distinct from, for instance, the individuals who have chosen to leave such institutions for a range of reasons or who have succumbed to the oppressive hierarchical regimes of power in academia and become a total conformist. An 'outsider within' attempts to 'conserve the creative tension of outsider within status by encouraging and institutionalizing outsider within ways of seeing' (Hill Collins, 1986, 29).

Therefore, the position of an 'outsider within' is not specific to only Black feminist academics, as it can be ascribed to any group of marginalized outsiders who encounter the dominant discourse of the powerful insider community. The term 'strategic outsider,' which is inspired by Hill Collins' notion of the outsider within, has helped me understand my own positionality—as well as many experiences like mine—in challenging the power differentials within and beyond the institutions to which I belong. 'Toxicity' is another useful concept that has been employed descriptively and metaphorically to depict the harsh reality of various structures of power. The former application of the concept concerns the literal medical materiality of the toxin and its effects and affectivities on a body, while the latter is an adjectival use of the term that illustrates how a dominant structure is harmful to the bodies of certain marginalized individuals. With this text, I aim to reveal how the strategic outsider can be an affective mixture of an intoxicated body by creatively reclaiming toxicities and remaining always 'bitterly' critical of a society that neutralizes forms of toxicity and actively justifies their harmful exclusionary impacts.

Analena Hope, a scholar and activist who is committed to working for communities of color, has referred to academia as a site in which the manifestations of 'toxic' society are evident. She has emphasized that academic spaces of knowledge production 'can generate stressors with the same corporeal manifestations as exposure to material hazards. [...] [A] cough, a lump, chronic headaches or fatigue, or the all-too-common academic feelings of insecurity, isolation, inadequacy and depression' (Hope, 2012). Furthermore, she demands that we 'begin to address the ways that the impacts of a toxic society are borne upon our bodies and psyches' (Hope, 2012).

Notably, the cultural and discursive quality of toxicity is also discussed in the work of another scholar, Gloria Wekker. In her influential work *White Innocence: Paradoxes of Colonialism and Race* (2016), Wekker explains how the pervasiveness of racial and 'discursive and organizational principles' has remained 'frozen, immobile, invisible and thus not discussed' (51) in the fields of knowledge production and policy-making practices with regard to women of color, migrants, and refugees. She states, 'in none of the prolific literature on women's or ethnic minority policy have I ever seen a discussion or even a mention of the toxic substructures upholding the worlds of policy making and academic knowledge production' (51). Nevertheless, Wekker does not dissect the precise meaning of the term 'toxic substructures'—she employs the term 'toxic' only five times in the whole book and uses the term 'toxic substructures' just once (in the chapter 'The House That Race Built').

Although she engages with the term implicitly, she understands a 'toxic substructure' as an underlying layer of the dominant order that governs academic spheres, as well as other institutional authorities, with the effect of silently excluding marginalized communities. First, Wekker (2016) outlines that she is interested in the 'silent and seemingly innocuous discursive patterns at the background of and simultaneously at the heart of these bureaucratic organizations, which both, among many other issues, direct their attention at women and blacks, migrants and refugees' (50). Then, she refers to 'silent patterns' as part of the 'cultural archive' (50). She focuses her critical lens mainly on race and elaborates on how racism operates silently through the open celebration of its 'nonexistence' in the Netherlands.

On the other hand, Wekker (2016) examines 'knowledge production about women and ethnic minorities in the sphere of the academy' (51). She further exemplifies how the toxic heritage has excluded women and communities of color. This argument links to Hill Collins' notion of the outsider within, which conveys that women of color are always rendered as outsiders in relation to their white colleagues. Wekker (2016) similarly states:

> While 'women' (i.e., white women) are the norm, the distance to them decides the location of other women, and they are again subdivided into allochthonous and Third World women. Culturally determined blind spots lead to this hierarchical, colonial division of labor: We are dealing here with a toxic heritage, the epistemic violence of a colonial discourse in which white people have silently and self-evidently assigned themselves a normative and superior position, the teleological axis or endpoint of development, and other women are always already located in relation to them. (62–63)

Here, a key point is Wekker's recognition that, within organizational policy, the emancipation of women is directed only at so-called 'allochthonous women (i.e., women coming from elsewhere, black, migrant, and refugee women)' (61). The term 'allochthonous' is the Dutch word for outsiders—those who come from elsewhere. Wekker observes a homogenizing act of differentiating between white women and all other women from different contexts, who are the 'outsiders.' Arguably, Wekker (2016) views the toxic substructure as central to the placement of marginal bodies outside of policy-making decisions and academic knowledge production.

In the second part of the chapter, Wekker presents a vignette about her teaching experience at Utrecht University that recounts how she was assigned to instruct a course on black critique. She frames this offer as an act of exclusion since she, as a gender studies scholar, wished to teach one of her preferred subjects, such as 'the construction of female subjectivities,' and the assignment excluded her from 'the caravan of women's studies,' which 'consisted of the thoughts and theories of white women' (66). Although she only briefly addresses her experience of teaching at Utrecht University, her account suggests that it was a toxic experience that, at times, rendered her an outsider.

Sometime after encountering that *only*, we read works by Wekker and others for our course 'Theory and Critical Research.' Engaging with this literature was healing for me; it validated that I was not alone and that I had also been experiencing toxins in my body: the body of an early researcher of color from the 'outside' (Middle East) attending on a European scholarship. I realized that, like Wekker and Hill Collins, I had been experiencing the feeling of being an 'imaginary outsider' who is 'seeking her bearings in an unfamiliar system' (Wekker, 2016, 67). I discovered a valid explanation for my 'over'-sensitivity to 'little words.' I felt the same since, as Wekker states, toxic substructures within and beyond academia undeniably exist in various forms, and have not been adequately addressed.

Still, my experience is surely not identical to those of other people of color in academia, and there is a need for more stories, visibilities, vulnerabilities, and critique to emerge. By sharing parts of my story as a GEMMA researcher in Western Europe, I do not intend to generalize; rather, I seek to highlight and validate my feelings about specific moments, which certainly extend beyond the example above. My expectations of my beloved gender studies program and my classmates have always been high, and we critically discussed (and resolved) these issues together on occasion, but these affirmative anticipations are exactly why I do not want to deprive those feelings of articulation or critique. With my story, I have attempted to demonstrate the need to seriously challenge the emphasis on hierarchizing divides between researchers or individuals on the basis of bureaucratic labels, nationality, class, and other factors. These seemingly trivial divisions can create feelings of exclusion among those who are exposed to them, and I believe they will eventually further materialize binary thinking in spaces that are meant to challenge various ways of binary thinking/making.

In addition, because of my education in gender studies, I understand that those little *onlys* matter, and I recognize that it is crucial to articulate such details and feelings of exclusion. Accordingly, I am not 'making a fuss' over 'little words.' After all, it was not simply a 'little word' that led me to realize my essentially outsider position while studying and living in Western Europe; there were many more moments in and beyond the classroom, on the campus, in my search for housing, during graduation, in job-seeking, and while trying to survive the cruelty of a pandemic. Reflecting on each of these moments would require more space than is available in this short piece. In brief, my experience of being a non-European woman of color in Western academia and its post-graduation (non-)academic job market has been intersectional. After graduation, those of us who were non-white, non-European, without a proper work visa, or not wealthy could only stay in the Netherlands or Europe by accepting irrelevant jobs, struggling with overwhelming anxiety while seeking employment, and applying for visas and visa extensions before and during the global pandemic, which further increased the precarity of the situation for many of us.

Of those numerous experiences, one incident provokes a particularly bitter response in me. During the pandemic lockdown and border closures, the expiry date for my post-graduation job-searching visa in the Netherlands was approaching. Since I still had not received my other visa or job application results, I had to visit the migration office in the city of Utrecht, where I was living, to ask the officer to extend my permit for just two to three months. I brought along all of my documents, including my degree certificate; however, immediately after I mentioned the word 'extension,' the officer stated that there is absolutely no way to request a visa extension, as it would be rejected. I patiently explained my complicated and precarious situation: that I urgently needed to remain in the Netherlands for two to three more months until I could move to my next academic destination. He then looked at my degree and documents, gave me the most petulant 'little smile' I had ever received in my life, and said, 'your extension request will be surely rejected, just like many other students' similar to your situation; but now that you have to stay in the Netherlands, you can apply for asylum status in the Netherlands and then cancel your asylum application if you don't need it later.'

He said this with full knowledge that the process of applying for asylum and cancelling it later is neither easy nor desirable and would force me into a more precarious situation and endless loop of vulnerability. Nevertheless, he could recommend it because he was a migration officer—the embodiment of 'toxic substructures' at their most extreme. For representatives of such unjust systems, there is no 'in-betweenness'; there is either the image of total victimhood, which they utilize to depict and dehumanize people, or there are people who are wealthy and privileged enough to enjoy freedom of movement whenever they want. Thus, the officer intentionally sought to lead me to the 'dead end' of becoming more victimized by the unequal Dutch system.

I vividly remember my frustration and indignation in that moment. I collected my documents and immediately left that dark office. Despite already feeling empty and frustrated, I decided to resist his 'little smile' by fighting harder. Although I was devastated, I was determined not to relent in the face of 'little smiles' and *onlys* and to instead further embrace my in-betweenness and my intoxicated, unwanted body. I became a 'sticky *allochtoon*' to the Dutch system and, with the help of my lawyer and the advice of wonderful people, managed to stay in the Netherlands until I departed for my next academic destination. After this experience, I have been fully aware of 'little smiles' and *onlys*, and will continue to challenge these numerous injustices of any size by drilling more holes, taking more hands, creating feminist kinship ties, and remaining persistent. The unjust system and multitude of exclusionary interactions that represent it want to deprive me of my dignity and either force me into silent obedience to imposed roles or heartlessly shove me out of the way. Thus, I actively claim the position of a stubborn *allochtoon* in Western society and academia—a strategic outsider—and fight critically as much as I can.

As Hope (2012) has explained, 'many of us entered the academy with intentions to address and somehow rectify the legacies of oppression plaguing our communities, and in doing so we have ironically become susceptible to the same precarious conditions we wish to amend' (2012). To avoid succumbing to such a vicious cycle, we need to constantly remain alert and critical of the same patterns that cause our precarity, regardless of where and when they arise. All of this anxiety, sensitivity, vulnerability, and uncertainty has prompted me to reflect further on the strategic approach to addressing the unequal 'toxic substructures' and 'brick walls' that have existed—and will probably continue to exist—in and outside of academia, as well as to re-imagine 'tools to break through the impasse that we [are in many ways] stuck in' (Wekker, 2016, 52). Again, I believe that one such tool is the positionality of the strategic outsider. The strategic outsider mirrors the figure of an informed, critical archiver who, as Wekker and others have perfectly illustrated, challenges the normalized, often invisible, and silent exclusions that occur at multiple levels.

In addition, in her account of neoliberal academia, Rosalind Gill (2009) uses the notion of toxicity to specify the shame and pressure imposed by academic failures in and beyond academia, and she emphasizes that such failures result from 'toxic conditions of neoliberal academia' (51). For Gill, toxicity is a fatal bacterium; it is a shameful feeling that is constantly produced by these toxic conditions. I argue that this toxicity can be reclaimed by remaining strategically critical of discourses and institutions that try to exhaust us into not thinking critically, not creating, and not finding allies. I have long been aware of these discourses, moments, and structures; however, I have decided to fight from within, as an outsider, while being inside—a contradictory position that I have embraced. A strategic outsider embraces the contradictions of institutions while non-exhaustively challenging their unjust mechanisms. Instead of merely describing or neutrally addressing the mechanisms of dominant ideologies as 'toxic,' the strategic outsider can 'willingly uptake' and embody toxicity and, hence, actively reshape, reclaim, and redefine it.

I find it important to acknowledge that, overall, my memorable years in the GEMMA program in Dutch (and partly Spanish) academia provided me with numerous beautiful moments as well as a chosen family of passionate and critical minds. I finished the GEMMA program with an MA degree with distinction (*cum laude*) and started a PhD on yet another prestigious fellowship at a renowned Western academic institution. Now, I am a Marie Skłodowska-Curie early-stage researcher at the University of Gothenburg, where I, together with a team of researchers and scholars, investigate the nature of hate (speech), its online/offline dynamics, and ways to counter it. This project is only the beginning for me, and it offers an opportunity to continue my research while remaining critical of certain toxic substructures—wherever they are located—and creating collectives by grasping more moments of solidarity and companionship with beautiful allies-in and outside of academia. My dream and determination are to continue to challenge and seek allies from within substructures, and never get exhausted.

# Works cited

Sara Ahmed, *Living a Feminist Life* (Duke University Press, 2017). https://doi.org/10.1215/9780822373377

Rosalind Gill, 'Breaking the silence: The hidden injuries of neo-liberal academia,' in *Secrecy and Silence in the Research Process: Feminist Reflections*, edited by Róisín Ryan-Flood and Rosalind Gill, 39–55 (Routledge, 2009). https://doi.org/10.4324/9780203927045

Patricia Hill Collins, 'Learning from the outsider within: The sociological significance of black feminist thought,' *Social Problems* 33/6 (December 1986): s14–s32.

Analena Hope, 'Can I live?', *Feministwire* (October 29, 2012), https://thefeministwire.com/2012/10/can-i-live/

GEMMA. 'Programme and calendar,' https://masteres.ugr.es/gemma/pages/programa

Gloria Wekker, *White Innocence: Paradoxes of Colonialism and Race* (Duke University Press, 2016). https://doi.org/10.1215/9780822374565

# 21. 'Who Deserves a Chair?' Performative Kinships and Microaggressions in the European Academy

*Ladan Rahbari*

I used to go to a lot of conferences. As my former roommate—who will remain anonymous—used to say, it seemed like this was a way for me to compensate for all the years I could not travel to/in Europe because I had no way of entry to European territory or its academic institutions before migrating. My roommate did not say this out of pity or judgement, but because she knew what it meant to be allowed to move around. She had gained similar advantages by temporarily moving to Europe, but for her, crossing borders had become such a stressful exercise that she just wanted to stay put unless she was forced to do so. Nothing made her more upset than the holiday season when our European colleagues talked about moving around the world, with no worry about visas and only caring about where they would have most 'fun' for the lowest price: 'price-for-performance,' as a German colleague put it.

I am not attending as many conferences abroad anymore. I try to stick to the local ones. I am at a bilingual Dutch-English conference in a Belgian university at the time of writing, and they serve all kinds of sandwiches for lunch. The vegetarian options, to my despair, all contain some kind of green pesto, which my digestive system cannot handle. I have decided not to eat them, and this has become a reason to have

https://doi.org/10.11647/OBP.0331.21

a conversation about meat with two European academics who are not vegetarians.

There are many vegetarians in my new home country, Belgium. There are also more seasonal vegetarian types and part-time vegetarians who occasionally go for large pieces of steak 'to connect with the hunter-gatherer they have inside.' I get irritated when people talk about hunter-gatherers to justify their 2019 lifestyle. Some detox enthusiasts eat meat for a while and then fast it out with juices that supposedly cleanse the flesh and stench of death out of their bodies. They are, of course, doing more than the full-time meat-eaters, in my opinion. It is a worthy effort, no matter what the extent. Still, even those seasonal animal lovers in Belgium may consume more meat in their meat-eating periods than a constant meat eater does in Iran.

That is why I find this conversation that I am having at the lunch table with the two Belgian academics quite absurd. I get asked whether people eat a lot of meat in my 'country of origin.' They have already asked me where I am from, and I have already told them that I live in Belgium, but I come from Iran. So, I am not sure why they do not just say Iran and instead repeatedly say 'your country' or 'country of origin.' I try to explain to them that, on average, an Iranian consumes much less meat than a Belgian. They protest, 'surely this must be wrong. You do not have vegetarians there. We have so many vegetarians in Belgium.' They confirm each other by nodding with confidence. The 'you' and the 'we' have a funny ring in my ears. I answer that even though I am a vegetarian, that does not make me an expert on meat consumption, so I would not be able to give them correct statistics. All I know is that vegetarianism is not the only factor that matters, and the average per capita meat consumption in Belgium is higher than in Iran. I have checked the data on this before because I am constantly asked why I, 'as an Iranian,' have become a vegetarian. I invite them to check the data. 'You probably became a vegetarian here, didn't you?' they say. I tell them my story in brief: No. I have been a vegetarian for a long time. I ate meat in my teens under family pressure. 'Your bones will be empty!' Nanah used to say to scare me. My family managed to feed me meat from time to time. I went back to being a vegetarian soon after realizing that the odds of bone diseases were not that much more favorable to meat-eaters. 'We will all die of empty bones one day,' I teased Nanah. I was ready to take the chance, even if 'science' was not yet as clear as it is today about a purely vegetarian diet.

The colleagues at the coffee table do not look convinced about what I tell them. They stare at my hands and my clothes. Then they avoid eye contact with me. They are suspicious of my words. My story does not fit how I look, or perhaps their grand narrative of meat-loving and devouring Middle Easterners. I must have been making these things up. They then slowly drift away, like dead pieces of wood floating on the water. In a similar situation, in their shoes, I would have politely protested or just excused myself. What is so hard about disbelief and conflict that scares people away like that?

I pick a panel to attend and sit in the back in case I find something catchier in the program. I need to remember to network, too. Networking has become a buzzword in academia these days. I never thought that it would happen to this extent. The conferences are turning into card exchange rituals. Every time I go somewhere, I end up gathering cards that I will hold on to for a few days and then dispose of later, feeling guilty and bitter because I cannot even remember which cards belong to who. Sitting in these panels, all I can think of is my less conventional academic writing, like this piece. I have been thinking about how my unconventional writing will be received if it is published. Is it going to be viewed as too emotional? Too subjective? I feel the shadow of the ruler of 'science' above my head. How many people will accuse me of playing the victim? Is it going to be judged for its literary, historic, or social value? Will my language be considered unrefined? I write in a language that is not my mother tongue, after all. Is it going to be received with an 'aargh! Yet another migrant story that we did not ask for'?

As others present their work, I drown in my thoughts until people start clapping around me. It is time for us to move on with the program, after a short coffee break.

I do not know anybody in the conference room, and I am not in the mood for networking. I pack my conference bag and follow the crowd to the coffee area again, a small hall with huge windows. One professor who gave a talk is now surrounded by people who want to talk about her presentation. I look around the room and see no familiar faces here either. The conference is bilingual, but I hardly hear anyone speaking English. I do not want to make anyone uncomfortable with my bad

Flemish. I pour a coffee into a yellow cup and head towards the small yard connected to the hall. The air smells nice here. I find a dry corner and put my heavy bag on the ground. I have carried my laptop the whole time, thinking that I would be able to do some work. Yet, all I have done so far is daydream.

I see another wanderer entering the yard. He turns in my direction, and we make eye contact for a millisecond. I am sipping my coffee when I realize he is approaching me decisively. He is coming straight towards me.

'We have not met,' he stretches his hands to shake my hand. I shake hands with him. He has a strong handshake.

'I just saw the program, and I saw this presentation about Iranian women. Is that your presentation? I would like to hear your talk,' says the man enthusiastically.

I confirm that it is my presentation. We then talk about Belgium. About the weather, the bikers, the train delays, and the language. We are both able to speak some Flemish, I learn. We say a few sentences to prove to each other that we can speak it. And then suddenly, he says:

'Let us speak some Farsi now!' in Farsi.

He speaks Farsi!

'You speak Farsi?' I almost shout in disbelief.

'Yes,' he responds with a glittering face. 'Farsi is my mother tongue. I am Afghani.'

This just became the highlight of my day. My mood changes immediately. It is one thing when you meet a new person at a conference, and it is a whole different thing when you meet someone who has the same mother tongue as you. This does not happen very often to me. I learn that the man's name is Iraj (pseudonym).

He tells me which city he 'originally' comes from. Suddenly, I realize that I am not as familiar with Afghanistan's geography as I would like to be. I cannot locate the city on Afghanistan's map, and I am ashamed of asking where it is. Is this shame legitimate? I try to ask a question to hide my ignorance. I ask him about his work here and if he is working on the same topic as me. He tells me he is not. He talks about his work and tells me that it makes him homesick to talk about it. He asks me something along the lines of, 'How can you not miss those landscapes of mountains and vast lands? The lands of warm people and strong hugs, where you leave your door open for others, so you do not make them feel unwanted. It is a different world.'

I am impressed by how passionately and poetically he talks about home and his nostalgia, although I am not entirely convinced we have the same image of our motherlands. I feel like he has a much more romantic image than I have. But that is the thing about migration: it is experienced differently and in so many colors. I do not stop him. He talks about different accents and dialects in Afghanistan, and I am embarrassed again, as I remember that I know so little about the country and its linguistic diversity. We must end the conversation and join the next panels, so we go our separate ways. Iraj will not present a paper at the conference, but he will join another panel as a listener. We will chat again later.

Sitting in the new session, all I can do is think of Iraj's face when he was explaining the imagery of his land—the land he misses so badly. I have never been to Afghanistan myself. It is a place that you do not wish to travel to if you are Iranian. Instead of thinking of traveling to all those close countries with amazing landscapes, diverse cultures, and people, you spend your time dreaming of Europe, America, and Australia. We learn very fast that we need to compare ourselves with the West and aspire to be like them. Nanah would say, 'we miss so much around us by gazing too far.'

I cannot find Iraj in the next short coffee break and then must go to my own panel. I hope to see him there. When I start looking for the panel room, I realize that the organizers have arranged a very small hallway at the other end of the building for the panel I am in. The hallways is not indicated on the building signs and is very difficult to find. It is a panel where 'foreigners' will present their findings from research on 'non-Western' countries in English, not Dutch. I have difficulty finding the hallway myself, and only manage to get there after being helped by a student guide. I see only a few attendees when I find it. 'Perhaps others will come later,' the panel coordinator announces, 'they might have difficulty finding the room.' There is at least acknowledgement that we have been given a lesser attractive space. It is not a room but a passage where some chairs have been placed, and people walk past us to go to the other panels. Our panel is the only English-speaking one at this hour, and since it might not be as busy as the others, the organizers decided not to waste a room. Charming!

The panel coordinator asks us if it is OK that we wait ten minutes. 'This is not an easy spot to find,' she repeats with a huge apologetic smile on her face. We all nod that it is ok to wait. We do wait, and after ten minutes, no one arrives. We then realize that the panel comprises the presenters and two attendees, one of whom is the coordinator. I hope every second that Iraj will walk in. But that does not happen. The coordinator has difficulty pronouncing our names, and every time she starts calling for the next presenter, she finds her experience of pronouncing the names amusing and bursts into hiccup-like laughs. We, the presenters, pretend we find it funny too and make eye contact with each other. She does not know any of us and gives no background information except for our university affiliation which she reads from a piece of paper.

When my turn comes, she calls me Ms. Ghaa-baa-ghee. I am used to mispronunciations of my name, as are many other academics with non-Western names. I understand that, most times, mispronunciations include very subtle mistakes that everyone can make. But we had plenty of time before the panel to let her know how to pronounce our names if she cared and asked. This was not a priority, and that is not a surprise to me. I keep smiling. Above that, while other presenters were called doctors, she calls me Ms. It is indicated in my biographical note that I have a PhD and I am the only woman on the panel, so this bothers me too. Yet, I keep smiling. I feel like my face is going to tear apart. I start talking for 15 minutes. And then, I answer some questions about my method. I am the last one, so the panel ends there.

The coordinator thanks us for presenting and leaves hastily. She must be relieved she does not have to speak English anymore or pronounce our weird-sounding names. I step out of that impromptu space. After so many years of studying, teaching, researching, and caring for social issues, I do not understand academia anymore. I have been negotiating with myself about this for quite a while. It has become such an impossible thing to understand: why do we do what we do? We have turned into a bunch of snobs gathering in closed buildings and discussing our idealism behind closed doors—a bunch of people obsessed with self-promotion and ignoring all the problems that our environments reproduce. We are not adequately connected with the world or with each other in these majestic buildings. It saddens me to think like this. This is the job I love and have dreamt of having all my life. I am looking around to find Iraj but cannot see him anywhere. It is a shame. I would have liked to speak Farsi some more. Suddenly I have a flashback to another conference incident.

***

It was one of the early years in Europe when I was actively traveling and conferencing. I was the first person to arrive in a conference room at an academic venue. I walked around the room to pass the time and looked out of the wide windows opening to a small and empty courtyard. Why do university buildings look so dull, I asked myself. So many wonderful things happen within walls, yet so little attention is paid to the aesthetics, colors, and comfort.

The room smelled damp, and I tried to find a way to open the windows, but there was no opening mechanism in view. A row of chairs and a table were placed at the end of the hall for the presenters. I chose a chair. It was not a special chair, but a chair perfectly identical to others. I made myself comfortable by hanging my coat on the chair and putting my mug on the table. I pulled out my laptop and started to go over my presentation to refresh my memory. Soon, I heard chatter in the hallways, and people arrived. A colleague saluted me, and I stood beside the window chatting with her when the fourth presenter, whom I will call Presenter A (A for anonymous), walked in. Presenter A was a European scholar who was relatively more senior than me. I remember that her work had received recent attention at the time. She declared herself with a loud and joyful hello, to which other people in the conference room and I reacted.

While still chatting, I noticed Presenter A took the seat I had already taken. Now, to be clear, the chair did not look like it was not claimed. The chair was drawn away from the table; my coat was already hanging from it. In fact, she had to sit on my coat that was visibly placed on the chair. My laptop was open in front of the chair and was connected to a charging plug under the table. I had a coffee mug standing beside the laptop. That chair was obviously taken. I did not think much of all this. I apologized to the colleague I had been talking to and walked to

Presenter A. 'Hi, I am sorry. I am sitting on this chair,' I said with a smile. I wanted to let her know fast to spare her the trouble of relocating with an open laptop.

Presenter A turned her head toward me, and there was a long pause and reflection on her side. She gazed at me for an uncomfortably long time before speaking. As if she was evaluating me and pondering on whether I was worthy of a reply. And then she said to me word by word and slowly as if she were talking to a child, 'As you can see, I am sitting here.' And then, with an exaggerated head gesture, she continued, 'move these things' [or maybe she said, your stuff. I cannot remember the exact words anymore], looking directly into my eyes.

I find it funny that my first reaction was to look around to see if anyone saw or overheard what happened or heard her. No one did. Everyone was busy chatting. I will neither forget the aggression in her voice nor the look she gave me saying this. She then turned her back to me. My smile froze on my face. What do you do in the face of such unexpected blunt aggression? I, for one, did not do anything. Before I could even manage to think about how to act, she stretched her arm in a rather dramatic way and with a slow rightward motion, moved all my belongings away from herself to open the space in front of her. I had to quickly pick up the mug, fearing that it would fall, and tea would spill on the table. She then dragged the chair she was sitting on closer to the table, but my laptop bag was on the way, so she pushed it away with her foot and tried again. The room was getting busier, and I was standing there in disbelief and shock. My laptop was pushed too far from the side of the table where she was sitting, so I went around the table to be able to reach my laptop and charger. Another chair was empty at the end of the presenters' row, so I walked there and placed my laptop. I then had to go back and gather my laptop bag from under her feet. And then I remembered that I had to go back yet again for my coat. The room was getting orderly. The coordinator was now standing behind the presenters' desk and waiting for everyone to take a seat.

'Sorry, but you are sitting on my coat,' I had to whisper to Presenter A. She turned and again gave me the same irritated look. As if my presence was an interruption or, better yet, pollution. She did not say anything but lifted half of her body to allow me to pull my coat from under her. This was a rather comical scene as she was not lifting herself enough, and I struggled to pull out my coat. I caught a few audience members watching us and smiling. I smiled back at them as I struggled to free my coat. I went back to my new chair and sat there puzzled and thinking, 'what just happened?' My mind was racing, and I was trying to make sense of her condescending gazes and uncomfortable pauses. But there was no time to reflect on all this. The room had quietened down, and the panel started.

I was so distracted throughout the panel that I did not even remember that Presenter A's talk was the one I had looked most forward to before arriving at the event. Ironically, her presentation was about academia, and she talked about toxic work cultures! I remember she put a lot of emphasis on being tired. The lecture received applause and praise from the audience. The Q&A went around her presentation as well. Someone mentioned 'sisterhood' as a way out of the toxicity; I do not recall if it was Presenter A answering an audience question or an audience member. When the panel ended, the audience went to her and congratulated her for the important work she was doing. I had had an internal struggle up until that point thinking of how she treated me, but I decided to be a good co-panelist and congratulate her on my way out. I waited for others audience members to leave. Presenter A was gathering her laptop when I went to her and said something like, 'that was a great presentation.' She raised her head and looked at me with a smirk, and then continued packing her bag without replying to me. This time someone saw the scene. I glimpsed at them but felt too embarrassed to make longer eye contact. I walked out, or better yet, fled that conference room, confused and feeling humiliated.

I met Presenter A years later. She was suggested as a speaker for an event I was co-organizing. She accepted the invitation to speak at the event, and in a few months, there she was. This time, I was part of the host institutions, and I was not an early-career scholar anymore. The experience I had with Presenter A taking my chair at the conference was by then part of a large inventory of microaggressions that I faced in academic spaces as a migrant, colored woman. Neither the experiences nor the gazes shook me as badly as they used to anymore. They did not become easier to bear either, but by then, I could place them and, as a sociologist, make sense of them. When Presenter A showed up at our event, she was still working on the same topic, which was, of course, extremely welcome within a hall full of academics. I enjoyed the presentation as well, but it has always been ironic to see academics making a career out of talking about how academia is broken and yet maintaining the same orders. Sisterhood came up again, and by then, I was already allergic to that word.

It was hard not to think about what had happened between the two of us a few years back. I was certain that Presenter A would not remember that incident, but as it appeared, she did. I learned this when two co-host colleagues, Presenter A, and I sat together to have food. This was the first occasion that we sat together during this event. My two colleagues went to bring us some sandwiches we had pre-ordered, and we stayed alone for a very short time. I decided to break the silence. After all, I was part of the host institution, and I wanted to be hospitable.

'How was your trip yesterday? Was it comfortable?' It was not just small talk. I had taken care of some of the bookings, and I wanted to know if everything had gone smoothly.

To my absolute surprise, she looked at me with the same smirky smile that I remembered from years ago. Then came the same long pause before she uttered, 'It was fine.' [or maybe she used 'OK.'] She then took her phone out and started playing with it. She had a 'do not bother me' air.

She had been so friendly until that point, and now, all of a sudden, after my Belgian colleagues left, she was the Presenter A that I had encountered at that conference years back. I still do not know what it was in her attitude that gave it away, but at that moment, it suddenly dawned on me that she remembered me. It is unlike me to try to talk to someone who avoids me, but I was reminded of the frustration I had felt the first time we had met. So, I decided to stand up for myself and said abruptly but in the friendliest way I could, 'we have met before, you know.'

Presenter A was holding her phone in front of her face. She did not change the position of her hand and the phone. She just tilted her head slightly and looked at me with a smile, and said, 'Oh, I remember.' She then continued looking at her phone's screen. My courage melted away, and we sat there in silence, waiting for my colleagues to come back. She, theatrically playing with her phone in an attempt not to talk to me. I, sitting still and wondering why this woman, this successful Western academic, has decided to dislike me. The colleagues then returned to us with sandwiches (including vegetarian options without pesto, this time), and Presenter A cheered their comeback and was friendly again.

While eating, Presenter A told my colleagues about her highly educated background. She said that professorship ran in her family, and she felt a sense of belonging in academia. She explained that her work and passion came from that. She was meant to be there and did what she did because academia was her home. As she spoke about herself, her identity, and her place in the world, it became increasingly clear from where her aggression toward me originated. That sense of *belonging*, the almost proprietary claim over academic spaces that had passed on to her and that she so proudly talked about, was not only about access to knowledge but also extended to chairs, tables, walls, and lecture halls. Presenter A was the one who embodied, owned, and deserved European academia and was deserving of choosing and sitting where she wanted. She was entitled to decide who belonged in those spaces and who did not. I could not sit in 'her' chair, let alone be her 'sister.' I was the intruder, the obvious outsider. I reeked of difference. Perhaps my foreignness leaked through my skin. My skin color, accent, and hair texture did not belong to the 'academia' she belonged to. Whatever it was, it was clear to her that I was misplaced, and she had 'recognized' me at that first glance. I was not the one who could take the chair. *She* deserved the chair.

***

I suddenly see Iraj waving and walking toward me. I am very glad to see him. We decide to go to a café nearby and have tea. I tell him how my panel went, and Iraj has his own stories about conferences like this. His name (his real name, that is) has also been badly pronounced, and he has been made to defend his research topic, something Western European scholars never have to deal with. We start by criticizing the way our research topics are pushed to the realm of 'area studies' because they are not conducted in wealthy countries. We continue exchanging stories. Iraj has worked in other European countries and has many stories of microaggressions. I tell him about my incident with Presenter A. We talk about the irony that 'sisterhood' and the performance of 'intimacy' and 'kinship' is coupled with microaggressions. And for the first time—after retelling the story to so many European colleagues who dismissed it as unimportant—Iraj is the person who gets it, empathizes with me, and does not attempt to reduce it to a mere 'misunderstanding.'

'We should call it what it is, and you know what? You should write about this experience,' says Iraj.

'Yes, I should,' I reply. 'Maybe one day I will.'

# Afterword: Reflections on Migrant Academics' Narratives

## *Umut Erel*

This collection of essays on the experience of being a migrant academic in Europe is an important piece of writing that comes at a time when there is more open and visible debate and reflection about the inequalities of gender and racialization within academia. There is an important body of research and campaigning work on the power relations subjecting racialized, women, queer and trans academics, and on their strategies for challenging them and creating alternative visions or practices of producing and sharing knowledge (e.g., Bacchetta et al., 2018; Gutiérrez-Rodríguez, 2016; Rollock, 2019; Tate and Page, 2018). Yet this work is uneven, and there is little work on European academia; this book is welcome in shedding light on the migrant academics' experiences in European countries. This volume could be a step towards building wider solidarities and strategies to challenge power relations subjecting migratized, racialized, women, queer and trans academics.

Reading the contributions to this book has felt at times eye-opening, at times shocking, and at times has triggered recognition. The experiences of migrant academics collected and shared here testify to the wide range of positions and positionalities in terms of migration status, migration trajectories, experiences of racialization, and gendered, racialized, and migratized working conditions.

Yet, in their wide range, each contribution also testifies to the entrenched and powerful mechanisms of migration regimes and working conditions, as well as migratized, racialized, and gendered professional hierarchies that are reflected in these accounts. Immigration legislation

     https://doi.org/10.11647/OBP.0331.22

often renders migrant academics more exploitable by institutions and individuals within them. Coupled with the widespread precarious working conditions that affect in particular early-career academics, this can create steep hierarchies which enable other forms of violence. Contributors to this book show how these structural inequalities have contributed to making them more vulnerable to racist and sexual harassment, and violence at the same time as silencing them. In this sense, this book is an important intervention into these power relations by creating a public space where these experiences can be recorded and made visible.

Some of the contributions speak of the conversations that migrant academics have amongst themselves, perhaps at the peripheries of conferences, perhaps in hushed tones. Unfortunately, these experiences are part of long-established structures and habits of discrimination and racism against migrant academics. Migrant academics often face the devaluation of their work. On the one hand, this is because they are seen as members of a minoritized group, who are also rendered as 'minors in tutelage' (Brah, 1997) and therefore not recognized as producing authorized or authoritative knowledge. On the other hand, migrant academics' own social positioning as at the margins of academia and of the national societies they live in can mean that their approaches to research prioritize critical, marginalized approaches to knowledge, which in turn challenge common-sense understandings of race, migration, and national culture—including national educational cultures—prevalent in academia and wider society. This combination of marginalized subject positions and epistemological approaches to knowledge production in the person of migrant academics can expose them to multi-pronged attacks on their credibility as persons, as well as the authoritativeness of their work.

Migration is often couched in terms of problems. One version of this problem approach to migration is that migrants are seen as *constituting* a problem for the societies in which they live and work—and this includes the institutions in which they work, the places in which they live, and the social and professional networks they are part of. Another version of this problem approach to migration is to posit that migrants *experience* problems—while it is clear that migrant academics experience problems, such as insecure, temporary, precarious employment, precarity due to immigration status, as well as a host of other issues related to gendered and racialized positioning, this problem paradigm itself can also have detrimental effects on migrant academics' professional lives and beyond. Thus, a number of contributions to the book recount experiences where migrant academics' expertise was questioned, challenged, or undermined, either because they were seen as too close to their subject of study, or because their academic and intellectual trajectory was devalued, especially for those from the Global South. While this points to the ways in which institutions and academic networks produce and reproduce hierarchies of what counts as authoritative knowledge and who is seen to legitimately embody it, racialized scholars and those from the Global South, as well as those from outside or the 'margins' of the EU, are only conditionally admitted to this group.

The chapters in this book also highlight the important role that gender plays in constructing hierarchies between academics and the knowledges they produce. A shocking (though sadly unsurprising) element in this is the way in which women scholars' work is delegitimized, and they are met with disbelief about their qualifications, skills, expertise. They are seen as sexually exploitable. There is a stigma that is attached to them when undertaking research, forcing them to find strategies that clearly highlight the professional context of research encounters, to protect themselves from the idea that their research is just another way of soliciting sex. However, they also encounter similar treatment by other academics at conferences or in the workplace, where they should be treated as peers. Instead, migrant women academics recount experiences of sexual harassment and violence in such contexts. This type of behavior builds on and exploits the privileges of white national male academics for building their own careers. But it is also a form of violence that actively builds and reinforces the gendered, racialized hierarchies between 'migrant' and national academics.

Alongside these interpersonal forms of discrimination and gendered racism, the contributors also outline the structural and institutional factors that shape their experiences of gendered and racialized working lives. This often starts before they enter the country with the difficulties of obtaining visas, then continues with the problems of getting residence and work permits. This is rarely a one-off process, but instead becomes a part of their working lives, as these permits need to be regularly renewed. The tediousness of this repetitive process is often accompanied by anxieties and insecurities. This process alone can be dispiriting and frustrating, yet it is often compounded by the insecurities of academic working contracts. Especially for early-career researchers, these are increasingly short-term and depend on external funding, which is hard to predict. These insecurities of working contracts and migration status further render migrant academics exploitable in a very competitive work context, where getting (or failing to get) a job, a publication, or a grant can depend on the strength of interpersonal networks or the good will of senior academics. Academic work requires considerable investment of time, energy, money, and commitment. Yet all this investment can feel like a gamble when there are few job opportunities, and those that exist often offer insecure working conditions. Much of this is part of the wider picture of neoliberal developments in academia, yet this book shows that this wider picture is clearly racialized, gendered, and migratized.

As some contributions point out, some of these experiences have been shared before, but this sharing mainly took place in the margins of conferences or intimate moments in the corridors of institutions. This edited book, in collecting and validating these experiences, makes an important intervention by challenging the exclusions, hierarchies, and power relations of migration status, racialization, and gender pervading academia. Such an intervention contributes to creating a wider public for these debates and hopefully seeds urgently needed solidarities to challenge these academic working conditions.

Reading the chapters' vivid autobiographical reflections brought back memories of my own. One of them is about working in a department whose ethos, proudly proclaimed on websites and conference proceedings, was one of social justice. Yet, when my colleague needed an extension of his contract to be able to extend his visa, it proved somehow impossible, even though the department was flourishing and attracting steady research income. My colleague, fortunately, was able to secure a permanent job elsewhere.

Another memory is of sitting through research presentations by colleagues who—without any irony or self-reflexivity—spoke of the participants in their research project as 'my migrants.' When challenged about the patronizing connotations of such wording, my colleague laughed. Well, I began to understand how engrained into the common sense of researchers such understandings of migrants as being childlike, needy, and dependent were when I heard her senior colleague's presentation. This senior colleague explained how difficult the economic position of some of the migrants she encountered in her research project was. Then she went on to spend half the time allocated to her presentation to sharing how she had bought a gift basket of foodstuff for her research participants and how grateful they had been.

Such framings of migrants as without agency, gratefully receiving researchers' attention and benefiting from their goodwill had been among the things propelling me to do research to challenge this narrative. Yet, years of study and training later, these framings continued. My professional positioning had changed, from being a student to being a researcher—yet, as a migrant woman, committed to challenging racist, sexist, nationalist, homophobic, and anti-trans, cisnormative knowledge production—I also realized that in the eyes of many colleagues I continued not only to be disruptive and challenging through my work, but also in my person. Many colleagues were heavily invested through their research in a narrative that presents migrant women as in need of rescuing, be it from migrant and racialized men, or from anti-migrant policies. They have carved out their own identities as speaking for these migrants through their research. So, to be faced with a migrant woman academic colleague can be a challenge. How could they relate to someone who combines these two identities of migrant woman and academic, when their own research and professional identity is built around viewing them as epistemologically irreconcilable: one is the knowing subject, the other the topic under study? The burden of making this contradiction bearable for our colleagues mostly falls onto migrant academics themselves, and the contributions in this book eloquently speak to this.

Another memory triggered by reading the contributions to this book is of a train journey with some academic colleagues. We were all in good spirits, chatting about work and other things. As the ticket inspector arrived someone from our group was joking that we might not have the correct tickets. I mentioned that I'd been on a bus recently that was stopped, with the doors locked, while police checked the residence permits. My colleagues looked at me in amazement, so I said 'yes, that was really shocking.' But instead of joining me in condemning such immigration controls in everyday places, targeting racialized people, my colleagues did not believe me. 'You must have made this up, they couldn't possibly check residence papers on public transport!' Other jokes followed about how I was perhaps a bit paranoid. I was stunned and tried to gather my thoughts to explain and 'evidence' that, indeed, such immigration checks were common. But as I was still thinking, I realized that my colleagues, all accomplished scholars who were well-versed in critical thinking, were averting their eyes from me in embarrassment and had quickly moved on to discussing another topic.

Years later, while reading Sara Ahmed's work on feminist killjoys (2016), I made more sense of this encounter. Ahmed analyzes how it is often those who name and make visible incidents, events, and structures that emanate from power relations and oppressions such as racism and sexism who then become seen as the source of the problem. They are seen as disrupting a convivial, happy atmosphere and, rather than engage with the issues these killjoys raise, colleagues and institutions often instead identify that killjoy with the problem, and they often experience being scapegoated and isolated in the institution. The migrant academics' stories assembled in this book are a powerful testimony to the necessity to continue this killjoy work of making visible and challenging the power relations affecting migratized academics.

# Works cited

Sara Ahmed, *Living a Feminist Life* (Duke University Press, 2016). https://doi.org/10.1215/9780822373377

Paola Bacchetta, Fatima El-Tayeb, Jin Haritaworn, Jillian Hernandez, S. A. Smythe, Vanessa E. Thompson, and Tiffany Willoughby-Herard, 'Queer of color space-making in and beyond the academic industrial complex', *Critical Ethnic Studies* 4/1 (2018): 44–63. https://doi.org/10.5749/jcritethnstud.4.1.0044

Encarnación Gutiérrez-Rodríguez, 'Sensing dispossession: Women and gender studies between institutional racism and migration control policies in the neoliberal university', *Women's Studies International Forum* 54/January-February (2016): 167–177. https://doi.org/10.1016/j.wsif.2015.06.013

Nicola Rollock, *Staying Power: The Career Experiences and Strategies of UK Black Female Professors* (University College London, 2019).

Shirley Anne Tate and Damien Page, 'Whiteliness and institutional racism: Hiding behind (un)conscious bias', *Ethics and Education* 13/1 (2018): 141–155. https://doi.org/10.1080/17449642.2018.1428718

# Authors' Biographies

**Apostolos Andrikopoulos** (PhD) is a Marie Skłodowska-Curie Global Fellow at Harvard University and at the University of Amsterdam. He is an anthropologist with expertise in issues of migration and kinship. His book *Argonauts of West Africa: Unauthorized Migration and Kinship Dynamics in a Changing Europe* is a revised version of his dissertation which received IMISCOE's Maria Baganha Award for the best dissertation in the field of migration studies. He has co-edited two special issues: one with Joelle Moret and Janine Dahinden for the *Journal of Ethnic and Migration Studies* (Contesting categories: cross-border marriages from the perspectives of the state, spouses, and researchers) and the other one with Jan Willem Duyvendak for the journal *Ethnography* (*Transnational Migration and Kinship Dynamics*).

**Tara Asgarilaleh** is a PhD candidate in the sociology department of the University of Cambridge, in the UK. Her PhD project is part of the Reproductive Sociology Research Group (ReproSoc) program at Cambridge and is funded by the Wellcome Trust. She was part of the Muslim Marriages project (funded by the European Research Council) in the Anthropology Department of the University of Amsterdam (2018–2019). She obtained a Bachelor of Science in sociology from the University of Tehran, Iran in 2014 and graduated from the Research Master Social Sciences (RMSS), funded by an Amsterdam Merit Scholarship, at the University of Amsterdam in 2017. For the RMSS, she wrote her thesis on organ transplantation and unrelated kidney donors in Iran, based on ethnographic fieldwork in Tehran. With her PhD project, she aims to examine how involuntarily childless couples, men in particular, can access and actually use assisted reproductive technologies (ARTs) in the socio-cultural, legal, religious and medical contexts of contemporary Iran. Through her ethnographic study she hopes to bring new insights into (in)fertility and men's perceptions of fertility and reproductive precarity in the use of ARTs in Iran and how this relates to dominant notions of masculinity.

**Vera Axyonova,** PhD, is Marie Skłodowska-Curie REWIRE Fellow at the University of Vienna, Austria, and Principal Investigator of the project 'Expert Knowledge in Times of Crisis—Uncovering Interaction Effects Between Think Tanks, Media and Politics beyond Liberal Democracies.' Previously, Vera worked in research, science management, and policy consulting, including as the Managing Director of 'Academics in Solidarity,' a transnational mentoring program for at-risk scholars at Freie Universität Berlin, Assistant Professor for International Integration at Justus Liebig University Giessen, and Hurford Next Generation Fellow with the Carnegie Endowment's Euro-Atlantic Security Initiative. Vera is co-founder of the ECPR Research Network on Statehood, Sovereignty and Conflict. She holds a PhD in political science from Bremen International Graduate School of Social Sciences.

**Olga Burlyuk**, PhD, is an Assistant Professor of Europe's external relations at the department of political science at the University of Amsterdam and an Affiliate at the Amsterdam Centre for European Studies (ACES). She holds a PhD in international relations from the University of Kent and has previously obtained Master's degrees in European studies (Maastricht University) and law (National University of Kyiv-Mohyla Academy). Olga's research interests are situated at the intersection of EU studies (with a focus on EU external action) and East European studies (with a focus on Ukraine). Her latest work includes book projects *Unintended Consequences of EU External Action* (co-edited with Gergana Noutcheva, Routledge, 2020) and *Civil Society in Ukraine Post-Euromaidan* (co-edited with Natalia Shapovalova, Columbia UP, 2019) and articles published in leading journals in her field (incl. *Journal of Common Market Studies, Journal of European Public Policy, The International Spectator, Hague Journal on the Rule of Law, East European Politics*, and others).

**Atamhi Cawayu** was born in Bolivia and grew up in Belgium. Currently, he is a PhD fellow of the Research Foundation Flanders, and affiliated to the Centre for Research on Culture and Gender at Ghent University, Belgium. Cawayu holds a Master's degree in sociology, gender, and diversity studies. In 2016 he won the DiverGent Thesis Prize for his Master's thesis on the educational trajectories of unaccompanied minors in sociology. In 2017 he was awarded a four-year fellowship for his project on the politics of child relinquishment, search, and reunion in transnational adoption from Bolivia. His research aims to centralize the narratives of Bolivian first families, and to bring the Bolivian adoption system into perspective. He relies on a feminist, decolonial, and anthropological approach to complete his research.

**Umut Erel**, PhD, is a Professor of sociology at The Open University, in the UK. Dr Erel's research employs an intersectional approach and explores how gender, migration, and ethnicity inform practices of citizenship. This has first been developed in her PhD, looking at skilled migrant women from Turkey in Britain and Germany (2009), then she explored these issues in the context of paid and unpaid work of refugee women in the voluntary sector and migrants in new areas of multiculture. Her current research focuses on migrant families and citizenship. This explores how migrant women's mothering practices can be conceptualized as citizenship practices.

**Sama Khosravi Ooryad** is a Marie Skłodowska Curie (MSCA-)PhD candidate at the department of cultural sciences at the University of Gothenburg, Sweden. She holds a Master's degree in women's and gender studies at Utrecht University and the University of Oviedo (mobility semester) under the GEMMA Erasmus Mundus program. She also has a background in English and comparative literature (BA and MA degrees from Urmia and Shahid Beheshti Universities in Iran) and is a published poet, writing poetry in Farsi and English. Her Master's thesis at Utrecht University was a critical conceptual study of the (feminist) online/offline protests by different generations of women in Iran.

**Norah Kiereri** is a fourth-year PhD student of sociology/anthropology at the Aix Marseille University. She is currently writing her dissertation on how divorced middle-class women in Nairobi navigate and negotiate local moralities to achieve and maintain respectability. Her PhD program is part of Project SALMEA: Self-Accomplishment and Local Moralities in East Africa, funded by the Agence Nationale de la Rechereche

(ANR-18-ce93-0009-01). Norah is also an enrolment management, corporate communication, and marketing professional with 12 years' experience. In her pre-PhD life, she served as Admissions Counselor at the United States International University-Africa and as Enrolment Manager and later, Associate Dean, Enrolment Management at the KCA University in Nairobi, Kenya.

**Karolina Kluczewska**, PhD, is a FWO post-doctoral researcher at the Ghent Institute for International and European Studies, Ghent University, Belgium. She received her PhD in International Relations from the University of St Andrews, in the UK. In recent years, she held research and teaching positions in Germany, at the Center for Global Cooperation Research in Duisburg, University of Marburg, University of Giessen; Russia, at the Tomsk State University; Tajikistan, at the Tajik National University; and France, at the University Sorbonne Paris Nord. Her research interests include development aid, welfare systems, and social policy in Central Asia.

**Emanuela Mangiarotti** (PhD mult.) is Research Fellow in the Department of Political and Social Sciences, University of Pavia, where she is also the module convener of a course on the history of India and Southeast Asia. She holds a PhD in international conflict analysis from the University of Kent and a PhD in sociology from the University of Genoa. Her publications and research interests weave together the political and social history of religious and ethnolinguistic minorities in South Asia, gender and conflict studies, and feminist theories and methodologies.

**Vjosa Musliu** (PhD) (she/her) is Assistant Professor at the department of political science, Vrije Universiteit Brussel (VUB), Belgium. Her research focuses on international interventions, EU external relations, and the way the EU creates and maintains its relations with its 'others' and how such practices also creep in in academic work. Her research interests also include post-structuralism and decoloniality. At VUB she teaches on international conflicts, international political economy (IPE), and European history. Previously she has been an FWO post-doctoral fellow and has worked as a post-doc at Ghent University and a lecturer at Kent University—Brussels School of International Studies. Over the past eight years she has been a visiting scholar at Warwick University, Pacific University of Lima, Marie Skłodowska-Curie University in Poland, and Dublin City University. Her book titled *Europeanization and Statebuilding as Everyday Practices. Performing Europe in the Western Balkans* (Routledge 'Studies on Intervention and Statebuilding') is coming out in 2021. In 2019, together with Gëzim Visoka she co-edited the edited volume *Unravelling Liberal Interventionism: Local Critiques of Statebuilding in Kosovo* ('Worlding Beyond the West Series'). She is also a co-editor of the Routledge 'Studies on Intervention and Statebuilding Series'.

**Lydia Namatende-Sakwa** is a Senior Lecturer and Coordinator Postgraduate Programs in the School of Education at Kyambogo University in Uganda. She holds a Doctorate in curriculum and teaching from Teachers College, Columbia University in the USA. She also holds a PhD in gender studies from Ghent University in Belgium. She has published widely within a qualitative, post-structural framework in areas of gender, curriculum, and teacher education.

**Ladan Rahbari** (PhD mult.) is an Assistant Professor at the department of sociology at the University of Amsterdam and a senior researcher at the International Migration Institute (IMI). She was formerly based in Ghent University, Belgium as the recipient of an FWO (Research Foundation Flanders) post-doctoral fellowship (2019–2022). Rahbari obtained a PhD in gender and diversity studies from UGent and VUB (2019) and a PhD in sociology (2015). Her research interests include gender/sexual politics, gender-based state violence and violence against women, political activism, and religion with a focus on Iran and the Iranian diaspora in Western Europe, and in the frameworks of post-colonial, feminist, and critical theories. Rahbari is currently affiliated with the Amsterdam Institute for Social Science Research (AISSR) and is the board member of the Amsterdam Research Center for Gender and Sexuality (ARC-GS), and the Amsterdam Center for Migration Research (ACMR). She teaches courses such as 'Migration, Race, and Ethnicity', 'Decolonial and Post-Colonial Perspectives' and 'Key Debates in Gender and Sexuality.' Between September 2019 and September 2020, Rahbari was the editor-in-chief of the *Journal of Diversity and Gender Studies* (*DiGeSt*). She is currently a member of DiGeSt's editorial board. She is also a member of Amsterdam Young Academy (2021–2026).

**Sanam Roohi**, PhD, is an International Fellow at the Kulturwissenschaftliches Institut, Essen, Germany. As a social anthropologist, her work straddles the themes of embodied migration infrastructures, transnational resource flows and their ramifications on caste-and-religious inflected community formations within the Indian diaspora. With a PhD in anthropology from the University of Amsterdam, her research outputs include the publication of a few book chapters and articles in journals including *Modern Asian Studies, Journal of Contemporary Asia, International Political Sociology,* and *Ethnic and Migration Studies,* apart from a co-produced film on diaspora philanthropy. She has worked as an Assistant Professor at St Joseph's (Autonomous), Bangalore between September 2016 and April 2018, was a 2018 SSRC InterAsia Fellow at the Global and Transregional Studies Platform, Georg-August University, Göttingen, and a Marie Curie COFUND fellow at Max Weber Kolleg, Erfurt, Germany between September 2018 and August 2020. Roohi is also on the editorial board of the journal *Comparative Migration Studies*.

**Bojan Savić**, PhD, is a Lecturer in international relations at the University of Kent at Brussels. Bojan received his PhD from the University of Kent at Brussels in 2012 and his MA degrees in European studies (University of Maastricht, 2007) and international relations (European Institute, Nice, 2008) before joining Virginia Tech's National Capital Region campus in Alexandria, VA as a post-doctoral researcher. His MA and PhD research focused on the formal modelling of intra-alliance relations, culminating in a doctoral dissertation on post-Cold War transformations of NATO's civilian and military structures. His current research combines insights from critical geopolitics, post-colonial studies, critical security studies, and international development. Dr Savić's new monograph on the legacies of 'global governance' in Afghanistan investigates how post-colonial subjects are produced and managed through population containment, financial and economic incentives, and racialized security.

**Maryna Shevtsova**, PhD, is EUTOPIA Post-Doctoral Fellow at the Faculty of Arts, in the University of Ljubljana, Slovenia. She is also a Senior FWO Fellow with KU Leuven, Belgium (2021/2026, start date postponed due to EUTOPIA fellowship). Maryna was a Swedish

Institute Post-Doctoral Fellow at the gender studies department of the University of Lund in 2020 and a Fulbright Scholar at the University of Florida, USA in 2018/19. Her most recent publications include the book *LGBTI Politics and Value Change in Ukraine and Turkey: Exporting Europe?* (Routledge, 2021) and edited volumes *LGBTQ+ Activism in Central and Eastern Europe: Resistance, Representation, and Identity* (with Radzhana Buyantueva, Palgrave Macmillan, 2019) and *LGBTI Asylum Seekers and Refugees from a Legal and Political Perspective: Persecution, Asylum, and Integration* (with Arzu Guler and Deniz Venturi, Springer, 2019). She is also a winner of the 2022´s Emma Goldman Award for her engagement in feminist research and human rights activism.

**Dragana Stojmenovska**, PhD, is a post-doctoral researcher in the department of sociology at New York University. She holds a PhD in sociology from the University of Amsterdam (2022). Her current research focuses on gender inequality in the workplace. Stojmenovska is the recipient of an NWO (Dutch Research Council) Rubicon grant for research on the stalled narrowing of the gender pay gap (2022–2024), and an NWO Research Talent grant for her PhD project on women's under-representation in workplace authority (2016–2021). Her work has been published in general sociology journals as well as in journals specializing in the study of gender and work (incl. *European Sociological Review*, *Gender, Work & Organization*, *Social Forces*, and others).

**Alexander Strelkov**, PhD, graduated in political science from the Russian State University of Humanities back in 2006. Afterwards he spent four years at the Institute of Europe (Russian Academy of Sciences), dealing with EU foreign policy, EU-Russia relations, and European neighborhood policy. Taking up an opportunity to do a PhD on national parliaments and EU integration, he moved to Maastricht in 2010, staying there until 2017, defending a PhD (2015) as well as teaching a variety of politics- and international-relations-related courses. Subsequently he has worked at Leiden University College and Erasmus University College, where he currently holds the position of Senior Lecturer in politics. Apart from scholarly work, such as publishing peer-reviewed articles (*West European Politics*, *East European Politics*, *Journal of Contemporary European Studies*, *Journal of European Integration*, *European Foreign Affairs*

*Review*), he has been involved in policy work and trainings with Aspen Institute and Clingendael. Alexander's professional interests have evolved beyond EU studies and international relations, embracing rule of law and democracy promotion, and currently shift in the direction of international political economy, anti-money laundering, and tax evasion.

**Mihnea Tănăsescu**, PhD, is a Research Fellow in the school of humanities and social sciences, service of sociology and anthropology, University of Mons, Belgium, as well as Associate Researcher of the political science department at the Vrije Universiteit Brussel, Belgium. He works in political theory and political ecology, focusing on the representation of nature, conflicts in nature conservation and restoration, and legal innovations in environmental law. His latest books are *Ecocene Politics* (Open Book Publishers, https://doi.org/10.11647/OBP.0274) and *Understanding the Rights of Nature: A Critical Introduction* (Transcript).

**Aslı Vatansever**, PhD, is a sociologist of work and social stratification, with a focus on precarious academic labor. After she got dismissed from her position as Associate Professor and banned from public service in Turkey due to her participation in the Academics for Peace campaign in 2016, she has been hosted at various institutions in Germany and Italy. Her ongoing research project at Bard College Berlin investigates forms of academic labor activism in Europe. Her books include *Ursprünge des Islamismus im Osmanischen Reich. Eine weltsystemanalytische Perspektive* (Dr Kovač, 2010), *Ne Ders Olsa Veririz. Akademisyenin Vasıfsız İşçiye Dönüşümü* (Ready to Teach Anything. The Transformation of the Academic into Unskilled Worker, İletişim, 2015—co-authored with Meral Gezici-Yalçın), and *At the Margins of Academia. Exile, Precariousness, and Subjectivity* (Brill, 2020).

**Martina Vitáčková**, PhD, is Guest Professor of Afrikaans literature at the Ghent Center for Afrikaans and Guest Professor of the study of South Africa, Ghent University, Belgium, working on contemporary popular romance in Afrikaans. She received a PhD in theory of literature for her thesis *Back to the Roots? Forming New Concepts of Women's Identity in Contemporary Postcolonial Literature Written by Women in Dutch and Afrikaans*. Furthermore, she co-authored *The History of Dutch Literature*, written in Czech (2015). She spent five years as a post-doc at the

University of Pretoria, where she co-founded the Gender Studies research group—GR@UP. Martina publishes on the topics of feminist literary theory, Afrikaans and Dutch literature, and most recently, popular romance.

**Anonymous contributor** (PhD): due to the sensitivity of the topic of mental health and other personal circumstances, the contributor will remain anonymous.

# Index

# About the Team

Alessandra Tosi was the managing editor for this book.

Rosalyn Sword performed the copy-editing, proofreading and indexing.

Jeevanjot Kaur Nagpal designed the cover. The cover was produced in InDesign using the Fontin font.

Melissa Purkiss typeset the book in InDesign.

Luca Baffa produced the paperback and hardback editions. The text font is Tex Gyre Pagella; the heading font is Californian FB.

Luca produced the EPUB, AZW3, PDF and HTML editions — the conversion is performed with open source software such as pandoc (https://pandoc.org/) created by John MacFarlane and other tools freely available on our GitHub page (https://github.com/OpenBookPublishers).

Sacha PG Tanna produced the XML edition.

# This book need not end here...

## Share

All our books — including the one you have just read — are free to access online so that students, researchers and members of the public who can't afford a printed edition will have access to the same ideas. This title will be accessed online by hundreds of readers each month across the globe: why not share the link so that someone you know is one of them?

This book and additional content is available at:

https://doi.org/10.11647/OBP.0331

## Donate

Open Book Publishers is an award-winning, scholar-led, not-for-profit press making knowledge freely available one book at a time. We don't charge authors to publish with us: instead, our work is supported by our library members and by donations from people who believe that research shouldn't be locked behind paywalls.

Why not join them in freeing knowledge by supporting us: https://www.openbookpublishers.com/support-us

Follow @OpenBookPublish

Read more at the Open Book Publishers BLOG

# You may also be interested in:

**Democratising Participatory Research**
**Pathways to Social Justice from the South**
*Carmen Martinez-Vargas*

https://doi.org/10.11647/OBP.0273

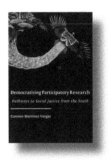

**Discourses We Live By**
**Narratives of Educational and Social Endeavour**
*Hazel R. Wright and Marianne Høyen (eds)*

https://doi.org/10.11647/OBP.0203

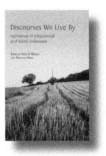

**Hanging on to the Edges**
**Essays on Science, Society and the Academic Life**
*Daniel Nettle*

https://doi.org/10.11647/OBP.0155

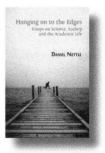

Printed in the USA
CPSIA information can be obtained
at www.ICGtesting.com
LVHW050008281023
762381LV00026B/417